Keto Diet for Women Over 50

An Essential Guide to Approaching the Ketogenic Diet and Losing Weight Effectively

CHAPTER 1: INTRODUCTION TO A KETO DIET 3

CHAPTER 2: ADVANTAGES OF THE KETO DIET 12

CHAPTER 3: KETO DIET FOR FEMALES OVER 50 16

CHAPTER 4: 7-DAY KETOGENIC KETO DIET MEAL PLAN FOR OLDER 20

CHAPTER 5: MYTHS AND FACTS ABOUT KETO................................31

CHAPTER 6: KETO RECIPES 65

CONCLUSIONS 122

Chapter 1: Introduction to A Keto Diet

A ketogenic diet is a high-fat, adequate-protein, low-starch keto diet that in medication is utilized basically to get troublesome control (refractory) epilepsy—this routine power the body to consume fats instead of sugars. Typically, the sugars contained in nourishment are changed over into glucose, which is then shipped around the body and is significant in powering cerebrum work. Be that as it may, if little starch stays in the eating routine, the liver proselyte's fat into unsaturated fats and ketone bodies. The ketone bodies go into the cerebrum and supplant glucose as a vitality source. A degree of ketone bodies in the blood, a state is known as ketogenic, prompts a decrease in the chance of epileptic seizures. Around half of the youngsters with epilepsy who have attempted some type of eating regimen saw all the seizures drop by at any rate half. The impact perseveres significantly in the wake of ending the eating routine. Some proof shows that grown-ups with epilepsy may profit by the eating routine and that a less rigorous method, such as an adjusted Atkins keto diet, is comparatively successful. Potential reactions may incorporate clogging, elevated cholesterol, development easing back, and kidney stones.

Different Types of Keto Diets
There are several different types of a keto diet, including:
1. The Standard Keto Diet
This is a very low-carb and protein, and high-fat eating schedule. It usually contains 75% fat, 20% protein, and just 5% carbs.
2. The Designed keto Diet (CKD)
This eating routine incorporates times of higher-carb refeeds, for instance, five ketogenic days followed by two high-carb days.
3. The concentrated on the keto diet (TKD)

This eating routine grants you to incorporate carbs around works out.

4. A High-protein keto Diet

This resembles a standard ketogenic keto diet yet fuses more protein. The extent usually is 60% fat, 35% protein, and 5% carbs.

Restorative Points of Interest of Keto

The keto diet began as a gadget for treating neurological contamination like epilepsy. Studies have now shown that sustenance can have benefits for a full scope of prosperity conditions:

1. Coronary disease

The keto diet can improve peril factors like muscle versus fat, HDL cholesterol levels, heartbeat, and glucose.

2. Dangerous development

The eating routine is, at present, is used to treat a couple of types of danger and moderate tumour advancement.

3. Alzheimer's ailment

The keto diet may lessen the indications of Alzheimer's affliction and moderate its development.

4. Epilepsy

Research shows that the keto diet can cause significant declines in seizures in epileptic youths.

5. Parkinson's infection

One examination found that the eating routine improved signs of Parkinson's disease.

6. Polycystic ovary issue

The keto diet can help in lowering insulin levels, which may expect an essential activity in polycystic ovaries issue.

7. Cerebrum wounds

One animal investigation found that the eating routine can diminish power outages and help recovery after mind harm.

8. Skin break out

Lower insulin in the blood and eating less sugar or arranged sustenances may help improve skin irritation.

Keto for Weight Loss

Ketogenic expend fewer calories are feasible for getting fit as a fiddle and cutting down peril factors for explicit sicknesses. While low-fat eating regimens are usually recommended for those wanting to shed pounds, explore shows that keto is, believe it or not, a superior approach than weight decrease as opposed to various weight control plans. Keto is a powerful and filling method for eating fewer carbs. You can get alive and well without following calories, which shields different individuals from adhering to different eating regimens. There are two or three reasons keto is more convincing than a low-fat eating plan, including extended protein utilization. Higher protein admission is profitable for weight decrease and metabolic wellbeing.

- There is solid proof that ketogenic eats less are helpful for weight reduction.
- They can assist you with losing fat, save bulk, and improve numerous markers of sickness.
- Numerous examinations have contrasted the prescribed low-fat eating regimen with a ketogenic keto diet for weight reduction.
- Discoveries regularly demonstrate the ketogenic keto diet to be prevalent, in any event, when total calorie admission is coordinated.

In one examination, individuals on a ketogenic diet lost 2.2 occasions more weight than those on a low-calorie, low-fat eating regimen. Triglyceride and HDL cholesterol levels additionally improved.

Why keto?

Another contort on extraordinary weight reduction is getting on in individual pieces of the United States. It's known as the "keto diet." People advancing the eating regimen state it utilizes the body's own fat consuming framework to assist individuals with losing noteworthy load in as meagre as ten days. It has additionally been known to help moderate the manifestations of youngsters with epilepsy, although specialists are not exactly sure why it works. Defenders state the eating routine can deliver fast weight reduction and give an individual more vitality. Be that as it may, pundits say the eating routine is an undesirable method to get in shape, and in specific examples, it very well may be absolute perilous.

How it functions: Bring on the bacon. This high-fat, low starch keto diet regularly implies eating less than 50 grams of carbs a day under four cuts of bread's worth.

The upsides: While the exact instruments are hazy, ketosis is thought to have cerebrum securing benefits: As numerous as half of the youngsters with epilepsy had fewer seizures after following the eating routine. What's more, some early research proposes it might benefit glucose control among individuals with diabetes. An up and coming investigation will take a gander at the ketogenic keto diet as a weight upkeep procedure.

The drawbacks: While the examination is energizing, there's next to no proof that this kind of eating is viable or safe over the long haul for something besides epilepsy. Besides, low starch eats fewer carbs will, in general, have higher paces of symptoms, including obstruction, cerebral pains, awful breath, and the sky is the limit from there. Additionally, meeting the eating regimen's necessities implies removing numerous solid nourishments, making it hard to meet your micronutrient needs.

Mayo's decision: While the keto diet might be prescribed for specific individuals with uncontrolled epilepsy, the high-fat substance, and particularly the elevated level of undesirable soaked fat joined with limits on supplement luxurious organic products, veggies and grains is a worry for long haul heart wellbeing.

History of a keto diet

If you've followed eating patterns lately, you've likely known about the ketogenic keto diet. This high-fat, low-carb technique for eating has spellbound mainstream society, and more individuals than any time in recent memory are pondering whether it will have any kind of effect for their wellbeing. For the following a month, we will distil the realities about the ketogenic keto diet into a progression of articles so you can leave away with a superior comprehension of what this eating routine guarantees and whether it bodes well for you.

For this first article, we're going to take a gander at the historical backdrop of this regularly misjudged keto diet and track its ascent in fame today. You will be amazed to know that the purposefully entering ketosis isn't new; however, instead owes its motivation to notable epilepsy inquire about finished just about a century back.

The Basics of Ketosis

At an essential level, the ketogenic keto diet is established in the possibility that restricting your sugar admission and devouring fats instead will place your body in a "fasted state" where it will consume ketones rather than glucose-bringing about better wellbeing for you.

The focal thought is that following a feast plan of 60-75% fat, 15-30% protein, and 5-10% carbs place the body in a state called ketosis. While your framework essentially decides to run on glucose (sugar), limiting your starch admission will make it feel that it's destitute, so it will produce an optional vitality source from fat to keep sending glucose to the mind. At the point when you limit your carb supply, your body begins to separate fat into mixes called ketones, which are an elective fuel source that numerous individuals accept has unique advantages for your wellbeing and weight.

A History of Epilepsy Research

While the term 'ketogenic' wasn't utilized until the twentieth century, there's a chronicled point of reference for fasting for wellbeing. Old Greek doctors upheld for confining one's eating routine to treat sicknesses like epilepsy and other medical issues, and fasting was viewed as necessary to a reliable way of life. Fasting is the primary epilepsy treatment recorded by Hippocrates, and it was standard practice across a significant part of the world for more than 2,000 years.

While the vast majority today start the ketogenic keto diet to get thinner or, in any case, improve their wellbeing, the eating procedure began as a treatment for epilepsy. The exploration story starts with the current primary investigation of fasting and its job in epilepsy, which occurred in France around 1911. The examination found that epilepsy patients who expended low-calorie eat less joined with times of fasting experienced fewer seizures and had less unfavorable wellbeing impacts from the condition.

Around a similar time, an American osteopathic doctor named Hugh Conklin started to prescribe fasting to his epileptic patients to assist them with getting their seizures levelled out. Utilizing a strategy that made epileptic patients quick for 18-25 days one after another, he flaunted a 50 per cent achievement rate for grown-ups, and as high as 90 per cent for kids.

There are five varieties of the Ketogenic Keto diet, which have been distributed in medicinal writing as compelling medications for infections that have a hidden metabolic dysregulation, for example, epilepsy, malignant growth, and Alzheimer's. The first Ketogenic Therapy, known as the typical Ketogenic Keto diet, or great Keto for short, was planned in 1923 by Dr Russell Wilder at the Mayo Clinic for epilepsy. All Ketogenic Keto diets are a variety of great Keto, which is the most severe, seen by it's the proportion of fat to protein and carbs, likewise called the macronutrient proportion. Exemplary Keto conveys a 4:1 balance, which infers that there are four areas fat for every one segment protein and carb. As the fat has a higher caloric substance versus protein and carb (fat has nine calories for each gram, while both protein and carb have just four calories for every gram), 90% of calories originate from fat in a typical Ketogenic Keto diet. In contrast, 6% originate from protein, and 4% originate from the carb. The primary distinction between the five types of Ketogenic Keto diets is this macronutrient proportion.

All Ketogenic Keto diets are high in fat, satisfactory in protein, and low in sugars. This mix changes how vitality is utilized in the body, changing over fat into unsaturated fats and ketones in the liver. When there is a raised degree of ketones in the blood, one is in a condition of ketosis, which has a statement of therapeutic advantages for the debilitated and reliable. Notwithstanding the macronutrient proportion, the recurrence of eating can impact ketosis. All the more explicitly, a training called discontinuous fasting, which lessens the window of time individual eats for the day, can help in getting and continuing ketosis. At the point when the eating window is abbreviated, the body is compelled to get to vitality from its fat stores as opposed to calories straightforwardly from the eating regimen.

Keto Diet Variations

There are five varieties of the Ketogenic Keto diet, which have been distributed in restorative writing as successful medicines for ailments that have a hidden metabolic dysregulation, for example, epilepsy, disease, and Alzheimer's. The first Ketogenic Therapy, known as the typical Ketogenic Keto diet, or great Keto for short, was planned in 1923 by Dr Russell for the treatment of epilepsy. All Ketogenic Keto diets are a variety of exemplary Keto, which is the most severe, seen by it's the proportion of fat to protein and carbs, additionally called the macronutrient proportion. Great Keto conveys a 4:1 balance, which infers that there are four areas fat for every one segment protein and carb. Since fat has a high caloric substance versus protein and carb (fat has nine calories for each gram, while both protein and carb have just four calories for every gram), 90% of calories originate from fat in a typical Ketogenic Keto diet. In contrast, 6% originate from protein, and 4% originate from the carb. The principle distinction between the five types of Ketogenic Keto diets is this macronutrient proportion.

All Ketogenic Keto diets are high in fat, sufficient in protein, and low in starches. This mix changes how vitality is utilized in the body, changing over fat into unsaturated fats and ketones in the liver. When there is a raised degree of ketones in the blood, one is in a condition of ketosis, which has a statement of practical advantages for the debilitated and sounds the same. Notwithstanding the macronutrient proportion, the recurrence of eating can impact ketosis. All the more explicitly, a training called discontinuous fasting, which diminishes the window of time individual eats for the day, can help in getting and continuing ketosis. At the point when the eating window is abbreviated, the body is compelled to get to vitality from its fat stores as opposed to calories legitimately from the eating regimen.

Way of Life And Other Factors

Ketogenic treatment incorporates something other than the keto diet. Healthful enhancements, electrolytes, hydration, and action levels are likewise key. People who are experiencing stomach related issues, for the most part, need extra help. This is the place an accomplished ketogenic pro can be amazingly useful. Checking ketosis is another significant part of treatment. Ketosis can be estimated by three unique techniques: Blood, breath, and pee. Blood readings are the most precise and dependable technique for testing. However, it is, likewise, the costliest. Pee strips give a reasonable choice. However, readings can shift broadly dependent on hydration. Breath screens have comparatively differing outcomes, and a higher section cost, yet, innovation is improving.

Think the ketogenic keto diet is directly for you? Converse with your primary care physician before receiving a ketogenic keto diet, or interface with one of our certified eating regimen experts to decide a game-plan that is directly for you.

Am I a contender for a Ketogenic Keto diet?

While the short answer is yes for most of the individuals devouring a western eating regimen, we ask you to counsel your general expert preceding doing the change to keto. The Charlie Foundation will furnish you with the data and devices essential to embrace the eating regimen, and joining forces with your primary care physician will guarantee the most remedial outcome.

Chapter 2: Advantages of The Keto Diet

Accomplishing a condition of ketosis can have numerous advantages from getting interminable ailments advancing execution. While the benefits are all around archived, the fundamental instrument of activity isn't altogether known. The eating regimen improves the capacity of mitochondria, the force plants of our cells, to convey our bodies' vitality needs in a way that diminishes aggravation and oxidative pressure. Through upgrading how our body utilizes vitality, we brace our bodies' capacity to battle a few illnesses just as take no the stressors of our cutting-edge method for living.

Is it a good idea to be on the Ketogenic Keto diet?

We at the Charlie Foundation accept that a 3-month responsibility to the eating regimen is a base duty to permit your body to adjust to the new fat-based fuel source completely. Since a great many people following a western eating regimen are not capable of processing fat, ideally, this period permits the body time to become "fat-adjusted," using keto dietary fat proficiently and adequately. There is a statement of keto diet plans that will empower a ketogenic way of life, and adaptability is one of the signs of the eating regimen that make it simple to embrace as a long-lasting device to upgrade your wellbeing. Our keto diet can assist figure with trip both the short and long-haul choices most appropriate for you and your way of life.

Perspective from Our Lead Keto dietist, Beth Zupec-Kania

In my 33 years of working with sustenance treatments, none approaches the noteworthy outcomes I've seen accomplished with ketogenic consume fewer calories. I had the experience with many individuals on the eating regimen, which has taken me everywhere throughout existence. Together with The Charlie Foundation, we have prepared more than 200 emergency clinics in ten nations.

The ketogenic keto diet was utilized in a few significant U.S. restorative focuses as an epilepsy treatment until post-World War II advancement of a new enemy of seizure meds became a standard convention. The ketogenic keto diet was practically wiped out in 1994 when a young man named Charlie Abrahams created hard-to-control epilepsy. His folks found out about the eating regimen in a restorative coursebook and took him to Johns Hopkins Hospital in Baltimore, Md. His seizures halted inside long periods of beginning the eating regimen, and he stayed on it for a long time. He is currently 21, remains sans seizure, lives without anyone else, and goes to school.

The family imparted their story to the media and addressed a large number of letters that followed. Charlie's dad, Jim Abrahams, composed, coordinated and created First Do No Harm, a 1997 TV film featuring Meryl Streep and dependent on a true story of another youngster who additionally became sans seizure because of a ketogenic keto diet. This started a flood in intrigue worldwide and prodded further research, demonstrating the viability of the eating regimen as a treatment for epilepsy.

The keto for epilepsy was found in 1921 by Dr Russel Wilder, MD, of the Mayo Clinic. At about a similar time, German natural chemist and Nobel laureate Otto Warburg distributed an examination demonstrating that disease cells, in contrast to typical cells, use glucose for vitality. (Late enthusiasm for this hypothesis has incited

The Ketogenic Keto diet: A Compromise from Fasting

From the start, these outcomes were terrific. Notwithstanding, there was one glaring issue. While analysts had evidence that fasting could control seizures, the undeniable entanglement was that fasts are intended to be impermanent. Numerous patients found that their seizures returned once they came back to their ordinary eating routine.

As different specialists started attempting to duplicate these outcomes, some tried different things with altered fasts that concentrated on disposing of starches and sugars, as opposed to confining all calories similarly. In particular, Dr More stunning at the Mayo Clinic saw that specific epilepsy patient had fewer seizures when their glucose was brought down from eating a high-fat, low-carb keto diet. He, therefore, made the ketogenic keto diet as an approach to copy the digestion that fasting produces.

The "Exemplary Keto" Approach

The reason behind going keto was straightforward: patients could be kept in a fasted state uncertainly on the off chance that they constrained their starch admission with the goal that their bodies consumed fat rather than glucose. Moving the keto diet proportion for fat expelled sugar from the circulation system and set off the body to expend a corrosive known as ketone bodies. Effectively following the eating routine persuaded the authority to act metabolically as though it was starving.

Another Mayo Clinic doctor named Dr Peterman gets acknowledgement for institutionalizing the eating routine into the "great keto" approach that is still followed today. Right now, specialists advocate for a 4:1 proportion of fat to protein and carbs. Although these proportions are always thought about the highest quality level, a 3:1 balance was likewise viewed as gainful. Generally, worthy nourishments for the ketogenic keto diet incorporated the accompanying:

Non-boring vegetables: verdant greens, cabbage, broccoli, cauliflower, peppers, and onions

Full Fat Dairy: yoghurt, milk, and cheddar items

Protein: meat, pork, fish, poultry, soybeans, eggs and shellfish

Nuts and Seeds: pecans, pistachios, sunflower and pumpkin seeds, and almonds

Fats: both creature and plant-based

Natural products (with some restraint): berries, avocado, rhubarb and coconut

In the beginning, emphases of the ketogenic keto diet, specialists underscored the significance of exact estimations for precise outcomes, implying that nourishment was frequently overloaded to the gram before utilization to keep members destined for success.

The outcome? An eating routine as viable as fasting for treating epilepsy that could be kept up for far longer. Presently in its subsequent century, the fundamentals of the eating methodology remain generally unaltered. Keto diets recommended that members devour one gram of protein for every kilogram of body weight, 10-15 day by day grams of starches, and top off the rest of their eating regimen with fat.

Chapter 3: Keto Diet for Females Over 50

Some portion of ageing involves a level of decrease by how we can work, yet it doesn't need to be disabling and segregating. This is, sadly, a sad reality for some seniors and older folks in our general public. The high-carb prepared eating routine frequently recommended for individuals of this age bunch isn't helping, either.

Instead of seeing getting older as deplorable, we can bolster more advantageous mental and physical wellbeing at any age through an increasingly legitimate eating regimen. Furthermore, in all actuality: there are numerous focal points of following a ketogenic keto diet for senior grown-ups.

Benefits of Following a Ketogenic Keto diet

Here is a portion of the ways being in ketosis and eating well ketogenic nourishments can address concerns frequently looked by seniors today:

Insulin opposition: Many residents in our public are overweight and managing diabetes. This is not funny at all, as diabetes can prompt things like vision misfortune, kidney infection, and the sky is the limit from there.

Bone health: Osteoporosis, in which diminished bone thickness makes bones delicate and weak, is one of the most well-known conditions seen in older people. This is because the nations with the most noteworthy paces of osteoporosis will, in general, have the most elevated speeds of dairy utilization. What's much better is to concentrate on a keto diet low in poisons, which meddle with ingestion, and is wealthy in all micronutrients instead of over-burden on a particular macronutrient (calcium).

Inflammation: For some individuals, ageing incorporates more agony from wounds that occurred at a younger age or joint issues like joint pain. Being in ketosis can help lessen the creation of substances considered cytokines that advance irritation, which can help with these kinds of conditions.

Supplement insufficiencies: Older grown-ups will, in general, have higher inadequacies in significant supplements like:

•	Iron: deficiency can prompt mind mist and weariness

•	Nutrient B12: insufficiency can prompt neurological conditions like dementia

•	Fats: insufficiency can prompt issues with discernment, skin, vision, and nutrient lacks

•	Nutrient D: insufficiency causes intellectual hindrance in older grown-ups, increment the danger of coronary illness, and even add to malignant growth chance.

The top-notch wellsprings of creature protein on the ketogenic keto diet can without much of a stretch record for fantastic wellsprings of these significant supplements.

Keto in Controlling Blood Sugar

As we've talked about, there is an association between inadequate glucose and cerebrum related conditions like Alzheimer's sickness, dementia, and Parkinson's Disease. A few factors that may add to Alzheimer's infection incorporate:

•	An abundance admission of carbohydrates, mainly from fructose which is radically decreased in the ketogenic keto diet

•	An absence of keto dietary fats and cholesterol which are bottomless and sound on the ketogenic keto diet

•	Oxidative pressure, which being in ketosis ensures against

•	Utilizing a ketogenic keto diet to assist control with blooding sugar and improve sustenance may help enhance insulin reaction as well as secure against memory issues that regularly happened with age.

Significance of Keto for Ageing

Keto nourishments convey a high measure of sustenance per calorie. This is significant because the basal metabolic rate (the ratio of calories required every day to endure) is less for seniors. Yet, they despise everything that needs an equal measure of supplements from more youthful individuals.

An individual aged 65+ will have a lot harder time living on lousy nourishments than a high schooler or 20-something whose body is as yet flexible. This makes it much increasingly vital for seniors to eat nourishments that are wellbeing supporting and infection battling. It can indeed mean the distinction between appreciating the brilliant years without limit or spending them in torment and misery.

Subsequently, seniors need to eat a progressively ideal eating routine by keeping away from "void calories" from sugars or nourishments wealthy in enemies of supplements, for example, entire grains, and expanding their measure of supplement rich fats and proteins.

Likewise, a significant part of the nourishment picked by older individuals (or given in an emergency clinic or clinical settings) will, in general, be vigorously prepared and extremely poor in supplements, for example, white bread, pasta, prunes, pureed potatoes and puddings.

The high-carb keto diet so broadly pushed by the legislature isn't best for supporting our senior residents and their long haul wellbeing. An eating regimen low in carbohydrates and wealthy in creature and plant fats are obviously better for advancing better insulin affectability, fewer occurrences of subjective decay, and generally speaking better wellbeing.

In a Keto Talk web recording with Jimmy Moore, Dr Adam Nally discusses how he has numerous older patients excelling on a keto diet. In light of the data talked about over, this bodes well.

Ketosis for Longevity

Regardless of our age, it's never an impractical notion to improve your odds of feeling and to work great for an incredible remainder. It's never the point where it's possible to begin growing, although the sooner we start, the better our odds of maintaining a strategic distance from the ailment. In any event, for the individuals who have spent numerous years not regarding their bodies just as they should, ketosis for seniors can fix a portion of the harm.

As we talk about ketosis for life span article, the previous we can start making changes that help healthy weight, glucose, resistance, and the sky is the limit from there, the more prominent possibility of having less torment and enduring further down the road. We're all getting older, and demise is, obviously, unavoidable. In any case, what we CAN control to a degree is the personal satisfaction en route. Individuals are presently living longer, but at the same time, we're getting more broken down by following the standard eating routine of the more significant part. The ketogenic keto diet can assist seniors with improving their wellbeing, so they can flourish instead of being wiped out or in torment during the later, long periods of life.

Chapter 4: 7-Day Ketogenic Keto Diet Meal Plan for Older

You are eating keto results in restricting your net carb admission to 20 grams for each day. In case you're hoping to amplify benefits like turning around type 2 diabetes or on the chance that you have a high weight to lose, the keto diet might be directly for you.

On the chance that you need more carbs and don't have type 2 diabetes or much weight to lose, an increasingly moderate low-carb keto diet may be for you. Moderate low carb is simpler to follow, yet it might be less compelling than keto, which means you may get increasingly reasonable outcomes.

Top 3 keto cooking tips

•	Mechanize breakfast: Choose one keto breakfast to eat each day, like scrambled eggs. Not ravenous? Skip breakfast and taste an espresso. This sets aside time and cash.

•	Streamline with me. Cook two servings the second serving for tomorrow's lunch. Freeze different parts for some other time.

•	Attempt no-cook plates. Cut shop meats, cheeses, and veggies to make a lunch. Here are some more.

•	Maintain a distance from keto influenza

Drink liquids and get enough salt, especially during the first week, to limit indications of the underlying "keto influenza." For example, a cup of bouillon each day can make a difference.

Best Foods for Your Anti-Ageing Keto diet

Although you can't quit ageing, you can remain sound. The initial move toward great wellbeing in your senior years is to eat right. "You should take care of your body to run as it should run. You must have great support," says Joan Salge Blake, EdD, a keto dietist and educator at Boston University. "You need to start treating the body as you do your machines and automobile and your home.

I am eating for Older women.

As we age, the bodies change - by the way they look, yet additionally by the way they work. It also takes more time for you to process your diet. You do not drink much water, so you don't feel as healthy as you used to. Diet may lose a portion of its taste, so you probably won't be keen on eating. You may make some hard memories biting, you may very well not want to cook, or you may be worn out on eating without anyone else.

When these things shield you from eating high, your once all around oiled machine begins to sputter. Talk with your doctor about any difficulty you have as you attempt to eat a solid keto diet. You might need to meet with a keto dietist, as well.

Keys to a Healthy Keto diet

You most likely know the rudiments of a solid keto diet - loads of foods grown from the ground, healthy proteins, entire grains, some low-fat dairy and sound fats, and less salt. A few nourishments are particularly useful for more seasoned grown-ups who need to eat more advantageous.

Water. It's not nourishment, you say? Consider it one. As you become more stable, you may not be drinking enough water as you don't feel parched as it once was.

"Water is so overlooked. Our bodies are, for the most part, Water. In case you're regularly got dried out, simply consider what your cells resemble," says Robin Foroutan, a New York keto dietist. "You can't think as unmistakably; you get exhausted all the more effectively, you don't endure heat too.

Blueberries. "Continuously flavorful," says Angel Planells, a keto dietist in Seattle, "and pressed with different antioxidants." Antioxidants - things like nutrient C and nutrient E - keep your cells stable.

Fibre. Fibre from nourishments like vegetables, entire grains, organic products, and vegetables assumes a vital job in your stomach related framework. It can help forestall or ease blockage just as lower your cholesterol, circulatory strain, and aggravation. That can prompt a more beneficial heart. Fibre additionally can assist control with blooding sugar levels and lower your odds of diabetes.

Greasy fish. Heart-sound all-stars like salmon, mackerel, and sardines are high in omega-3 unsaturated fats. They can be a piece of a solid keto diet. Focus on, at any rate, two servings per week.

Olive oil. You can utilize this as a substitute for margarine. It's more beneficial than some different oils.

Yoghurt. Unfortunately, the bone structure deteriorates with age. Calcium helps to slow down and keep it under control, and yoghurt is a good source. Take yoghurt with nutrient D, which encourages you to take and use that critical mineral. Yoghurt also digests your nourishment and also contains protein. Also, it goes well with organic products.

Tomatoes. These and different nourishments high in lycopene, a characteristic synthetic, can help secure you against malignant prostate growth and may help forestall lung disease. Cooked or handled tomatoes (in juice, glue, and sauce) might be more excellent than rough ones.

Red wine. Liquor may help lower "terrible" cholesterol, forestall blood clusters, and facilitate your circulatory strain. Chill out. That typically implies close to one beverage daily for ladies and two per day for men. On the chance that you don't drink liquor, however, don't begin.

Broccoli. Contain a wide range of nutrients and antioxidants, and broccoli is rich in fibre.

Nuts. Rich in omega-3, unsaturated fats (the right type), fibre, and protein, walnuts are the centre of a keto diet. Go for five 1-ounce servings every week.

The accompanying models equivalent 1 ounce:

- 24 almonds
- 18 medium cashews
- 12 hazelnuts or filberts
- Eight medium Brazil nuts
- 12 macadamia nuts
- 35 peanuts
- 15 walnut parts
- 14 English pecan parts

8 Signs of Poor diet

The correct nourishments in the perfect sums are vital to a long and sound life, and your body's needs change as you get more season. For instance, you don't require the same number of calories, yet you need a higher amount of certain supplements like nutrient D and calcium. What's more, as you age, your body may experience difficulty taking in and utilizing nutrients found in nourishments, like B12.

Along these lines, more established grown-ups don't generally get the supplements they need. It very well may be a smart thought to know the indications of poor keto diet so you can chat with your primary care physician on the off chance that you notice any of them.

1. Feeling Tired

If you need vitality always, it very well may be an indication that you don't get enough of specific supplements, similar to the press. Excessively little of that mineral can prompt frailty - when you need more red platelets to siphon oxygen and supplements to parts of your body. Weariness likewise can be a manifestation of some wellbeing conditions, similar to coronary illness or a thyroid issue.

2. Fragile, Dry Hair

Supplements like iron, folate, and nutrient C are significant for your hair. If you don't get enough of these through your keto diet, you may see some undesirable changes. Your skin likewise may be dainty and pale.

As it may, other wellbeing conditions, similar to an issue with your thyroid, can influence your hair and skin, as well.

3. Furrowed or Spoon-Shaped Nails

The poor keto diet can cause a few changes in your nails. Like your hair, your nails can get slender and fragile, yet there can be different signs. One is nails that bend like a spoon, particularly on your forefinger or third finger. That can mean you're low on iron.

Your nails likewise might be furrowed or begin to fall apart from the nail bed. Notwithstanding issues with iron, nail issues can be brought about by low degrees of protein, calcium, or nutrients A, B6, C, and D.

4. Dental Problems

Your mouth is one of the principal places indications of the poor keto diet that can appear. An absence of nutrient C can cause the dying, bothered gums of gum disease (gum ailment). You could even lose your teeth.

If you have false teeth or absent or free teeth, that can change your nourishment decisions. Poor keto diet at that point turns into a twofold edged sword: If your mouth damages and you have a problem with teeth, it's much harder to eat well nourishments. What's more, that makes it harder to keep your teeth stable.

5. Change in Bowel Habits

Stoppage can occur if you don't get enough fibre, found in entire grains, natural products, and vegetables.

6. Disposition and Mental Health Issues

An undesirable keto diet can assume a job in melancholy. It can influence a wide range of mental undertakings and cause you to lose enthusiasm for things you used to appreciate. You likewise may feel perplexed and have memory misfortune.

7. Pure Bruising and Slow Healing

On the off chance that you wound effectively, mainly if there isn't a conspicuous purpose behind it (like falling or catching something), your keto diet may be having an influence. In particular, you might be inadequate in protein, nutrient C, or nutrient K, which are all expected to mend wounds. Nutrient C encourages tissue to fix itself, and nutrient K is significant for blood thickening.

8. Slow Immune Response

Without the correct keto diet, your safe framework probably won't be as stable as it should be to the battle ailment. Perhaps the most significant supplements for a robust, invulnerable structure are protein and zinc, alongside nutrients A, C, and E.

Step by step instructions to Stay Healthy

The ideal approach to forestall these sorts of issues is with a reasonable keto diet of organic products, vegetables, lean proteins, entire grains, low-fat dairy, and more beneficial oils. Pick an assortment of these nourishments at every feast to get the nutrients and minerals you need. Furthermore, attempt to confine bundled or prepared nourishments and heated products that are high in saturated and trans fats.

Nutrient Essentials as We Age

The ideal approach to get the nutrients, minerals and different supplements you need isn't with a shopping binge at your neighbourhood drugstore. It's from nourishment.

A decent, adjusted eating plan - loaded with foods grown from the ground, low-fat dairy, heaps of liquids, more beneficial oils, vital proteins, and entire grains - ought to work.

In any case, numerous more established grown-ups make some hard memories adhering to a sound keto diet. There could be various reasons, as:

- Absence of hunger
- Inconvenience biting
- Fixed spending plans
- Inconvenience finding sound
- food and diet

As it may, they are not generally the appropriate response. Take nutrient A - significant for healthy eyes, skin, and insusceptible framework. "Nutrient An is to some degree a dubious nutrient since you can get harmful from it," says Ronni Chernoff, Ph.D., partner chief of the Arkansas Geriatric Education Collaborative.

A lot of it can cause queasiness, migraines, wooziness, and different side effects. She includes that more established individuals are bound to have those when they take an excess of because their bodies don't manage the nutrient too.

In the wake of chatting with your primary care physician, if you choose, you need a multivitamin and a total enhancement, one that gives 100% of the suggested measures of nutrients and minerals. Take additional consideration when you:

- Take more than one enhancement.
- Utilize an increase instead of drug
- Take them alongside with over-the-counter or doctor-prescribed medications.

"You need to ensure your left hand comprehends what your correct hand is doing," says Joan Salge Blake, EdD, clinical partner educator of keto diet at Boston University.

How Vitamins Can Help

More established grown-ups have various necessities with regards to nutrients. For example, the perfect measure of calcium can help fight off osteoporosis in ladies. Vitamin D, which enables your body to take in and use calcium, additionally forestalls bone misfortune and broken bones in more established grown-ups.

It's occasionally challenging to know precisely what you need. However, on the off chance that you have a decent keto diet, you're most likely doing OK. In case you're despite everything concerned, Robin Foroutan, a keto dietist from New York, recommends you inquire as to whether enhancements should help.

Before you go to the store, it's imperative to know the expression "supplements" incorporates nutrients and minerals, yet additionally herbs and different botanicals, amino acids, proteins, and different things. Some are alleged strength items like probiotics or fish oils.

Vitamin

Vitamin D. This supplement encourages you to take in calcium and phosphorus, so it's critical for robust bones and teeth. More established grown-ups don't make it also, so enhancements can help make you less inclined to have bone diseases and broken bones.

Vitamin B12. This is essential for keeping platelets and nerve cells sound. Ageing influences how well you take in and use B12 from nourishments, so in case you're more than 50, it's presumably best to get your B12 from enhancements and B12-strengthened food sources like grains, just as nourishments that are wealthy in it, similar to meat, low-fat dairy, and fish.

Folate. This forestalls frailty. Spinach, beans, peas, oranges, braced oats, and improved pieces of bread can have it.

Vitamin B6. This helps your digestion and safe skeleton. You can get it through braced oats and soybeans, just as organ meats and entire grains. Your body likewise needs these:

Nutrient C. Oranges, isn't that so? (What's more, red and green ringer peppers, alongside different vegetables and natural products.) It might help shield you from waterfalls, help wound mending, and conceivably bring down your chances of having specific sorts of malignant growth.

Magnesium. In addition to other things, it helps keep your pulse and glucose levels consistent. It's additionally useful for your bones. You can get it from nuts or spinach, and it's utilized to strengthen some morning meal grains. Specialists aren't sure how well it fills in as an enhancement. What's more, here are some well-known things you can discover in the enhancements path that you may chat with your primary care physician about:

Probiotics. Gut wellbeing is likewise significant for your resistant framework. A few examinations show that probiotics - living beings like those found in yoghurt - help forestall a few kinds of looseness of the bowels and simplicity side effects of the crabby inside disorder.

Coenzyme Q10. Additionally called coQ10, this is usually made in your body and found in most body tissues. It might enable your resistant framework to work better.

Melatonin. A hormone discharged for the most part around evening time, and it's accepted to assist you with nodding off. The science on it is promising.

Fish oil. At any rate, two servings per seven-day stretch of salmon and different sorts of fish with omega-3 unsaturated fats. In supplement structure, however, no investigations have indicated that it ensures against coronary illness. Omega-3s additionally may help with indications of rheumatoid joint inflammation.

Spices and Herbs That Can Help You to be Healthy

No feast or tidbit ought to be bare. That is the thing that keto dietitian Monica Auslander Moreno reveals to her customers. "Herbs and spices make nourishment more delicious while boosting your wellbeing," says Moreno, an aide teacher of keto diet at the University of Miami and a keto dietitian for the Miami Marlins.

Herbs, similar to basil, are the leaves of a plant, while spices, similar to cinnamon, are typically produced using the seeds, berries, bark, or foundations of a plant. Both are utilized to enhance nourishment, yet explore shows they're crammed with solid mixes and may have medical advantages. "That is because everyone is rich in phytochemicals, which are stimulating synthetic compounds."

Pick the Real Thing

You may have seen that a few herbs and spices are sold as enhancements (oregano oil or cases of cinnamon remove, for instance). Except if your primary care physician prescribes something else, "it's ideal for eating the herb or spice as opposed to taking it in pill structure," Youdim says.

She says there aren't numerous guidelines about enhancements, and there's little government oversight. So a case might not have the measure of something that it cases too, or it might have undesirable added substances.

"Nourishment is a military," Moreno says. We don't have a clue whether you get a similar come about because of accepting a single fixing as an enhancement."

Best Herbs for Your Health

In case you're new to cooking with herbs and spices, Moreno suggests attempting a squeeze at once to make sense of which fixings and flavour mix you like. Here are some champions to consider adding to your next dinner:

Cardamom. This sweet, sharp spice is in numerous pumpkin spice blends. It's known to calm an agitated stomach, and lab considers you show it might likewise help battle irritation. One more advantage? "Everything being equal, it is high in minerals like magnesium and zinc," Moreno says.

Bean stew peppers. New, dried, or powdered chillies will kick your nourishment. They likewise may support your digestion and assist keep with blooding vessels sound. One potential explanation is capsaicin, the exacerbate that makes them zesty.

Cinnamon. "Cinnamon is good because it's sweet yet low in calories and sans sugar," Moreno says. "Furthermore, it's anything but difficult to discover and not costly, and you can add it to nearly anything, including espresso and tea." The lab examines show that cinnamon likewise may help with aggravation, battle off free radicals that can harm your cells, and battle microscopic organisms. What's more, some examination proposes it might bring down glucose in individuals who have diabetes or are probably going to get the infection, yet different investigations don't back that up.

Cocoa. You may consider cocoa the critical fixing in chocolate, yet it's a spice with numerous wellbeing advantages. The cocoa bean is packed with flavonoids, which are antioxidants that have been appeared to support heart wellbeing. Flavonoids appear to assume a job in bringing down cholesterol and circulatory strain and helping keep your coronary (heart) conduits stable, in addition to other things.

Cumin. Utilized worldwide and known as a critical fixing in numerous Indian dishes, cumin usually is wealthy in iron. It might assume a job in weight reduction, as well. One investigation of 88 overweight ladies found that the individuals who ate somewhat less than a teaspoon of cumin daily while on a low-calorie keto diet lost more muscle to fat ratio and weight as those on a similar keto diet who didn't include cumin.

Garlic. This plant has a fantastic compound called allicin. The lab examines demonstrated that it might bring down your odds of getting the coronary illness. What's more, other research shows that eating garlic consistently may help with elevated cholesterol and hypertension. Be that as it may, to get the advantages, you need to slash or squash the clove: Allicin is shaped simply after the cells in the garlic have been cut or squashed.

Ginger. Truly, ginger can help with a furious stomach. "It has a quieting impact on the covering of your stomach related framework and can ease queasiness," Moreno says.

Lab concentrates likewise show that ginger has anti-incendiary and antioxidant properties and may assume a job in forestalling infections like a disease.

Rosemary. An ultra-fragrant herb, rosemary is wealthy in antioxidants that forestall cell harm, Moreno says. In any event, sniffing it might be beneficial for you. One examination found that individuals who got a whiff of rosemary performed better on memory tests and other mental undertakings, contrasted, and the individuals who didn't. Specialists think one about its mixes, called 1,8 cineole, may help mind action.

Turmeric. This yellow spice gets a ton of promotion and in light of current circumstances. It's a decent wellspring of curcumin, an antioxidant that facilitates irritation. Research recommends that curcumin may help ease torment. What's more, other research shows that eating even modest quantities of turmeric consistently may help forestall or hinder Alzheimer's illness, potentially by preventing the cerebrum plaques that lead to dementia.

Chapter 5: Myths and Facts About Keto

After 50, your body doesn't process nourishment how it did when you were more youthful. Your digestion eases back down, and you're bound to lose bulk and see changes in your weight.

Subsequently, it requires somewhat more idea and exertion to ensure you get enough keto diet and remain a healthy weight, says keto dietitian Nancy Farrell. "I'm not into telling others that they ought to maintain a strategic distance from explicit nourishments," says Farrell, a representative for the Academy of Keto diet and Keto dietetics.

Conditions identified with undesirable keto diets - like diabetes, weight, respiratory failures, and strokes - will, in general, happen all the more regularly as we age. So individuals more than 50 need to watch their calories more intently and eat less nourishment with included sugar or a ton of big fats, similar to the ones in spread or shortening.

Specialists state men more than 50 who are tolerably dynamic ought to get somewhere in the range of 2,200 and 2,400 calories per day. For ladies, that number is around 1,800 calories. Monitoring that is simpler since the administration began expecting cafés to post carbohydrate contents on their menus.

"I was simply flying back from North Dakota, and I went to a spot to get a sandwich to take on the plane," says Dawson-Hughes, an endocrinologist.

"The sandwich had 300 calories in it. One rare treat they were selling had 350 calories. If I hadn't seen those names, I would have snatched a treat alongside the chicken sandwich."

That is the sort of information that proves to be useful when you're attempting to remain sound more than 50. There are still a few misguided judgments out there that specialists are trying to clear up.

Myth: Since my digestion is slower, I have to eat less.

Not really, Farrell says. As you age, it might be more enthusiastically for your body to take in and use nutrients and minerals like nutrient B12, calcium, zinc, or iron. What's more, a few prescriptions can make that considerably harder.

Also, numerous grown-ups don't get enough nutrient D, which you requirement for bone and muscle quality. This usually is because they need more dairy in their keto diets, or they don't get out in the sun frequently.

That implies you may need to eat a more significant amount of certain things and less of others to ensure you get the correct keto diet. For instance, you may need to eat more protein and get more exercise to compensate for the loss of bulk, Farrell says. Or then again, you may require more leafy foods, Dawson-Hughes says.

Myth: I'm not ravenous at present. It's OK to skirt dinner.

There are advantages to keeping an ordinary calendar. "Your body is a campfire," Farrell says. "In case you have ablaze, you're going to toss another bit of wood to keep that fire consuming. That keeps the digestion fully operational. The caution is you must toss the correct quality and a pleasant quantity, not overcompensating either."

Fact: It's past the point where it is possible to change my propensities.

"I see patients who have significant ailments and incessant sickness expresses that are deteriorating, and they are looking to slow the procedure," Farrell says. "They wish they would have been progressively genuine about wellbeing and keto diet in their more youthful years."

Be that as it may, while it might be harder to change a few propensities, the more you've had them, "it is rarely past the point of no return or too soon to deal with conduct changes in any period of life."

In case you're stressed over your weight, go with nourishments that pack a great deal of keto diet without a ton of calories. These "supplement thick" nourishments incorporate foods grown from the ground, entire grains like oats and dark coloured rice, and beans and nuts. Lean meat, eggs, and fish additionally fall into this class, alongside low-fat milk and cheddar.

What's more, skirt the arrangement supper at your nearby drive-through, Farrell says. Sugary beverages or treats, nourishments made with margarine or shortening, or nourishments produced using refined grains, similar to white bread or pasta, pack more calories with less keto diet.

"Things that don't include any keto diet worth yet include calories will be fulfilling and cause you to feel full, and afterwards, you will get inadequate in supplements that are significant," Dawson-Hughes says.

Fact: It's everything about the keto diet.

The high keto diet isn't always about what you bring home from the store. At times the test is finding a workable pace in any case.

Loads of things can influence how well you eat as you age. Losing teeth may make it harder to surrender certain nourishments; for instance, or your faculties of taste and smell can be changed as you get more established, Farrell says.

"Warm chocolate chip treats new out of the broiler don't have a similar impact any longer," she says. What's more, a few seniors have physical issues that make it harder to get around, or they don't have transportation. Money related issues, sadness, or seclusion are increasingly regular as individuals age, as well.

Things Woman Over 50 Should Know

Arriving at 50 is an achievement; however, times can be upsetting. The children are most likely set off for college or are only moving out of the house, guardians are ageing, and you rapidly discover that your body doesn't endure what you put it through equivalent to it did a couple of years prior. This is an ideal opportunity to investigate your way of life propensities and cause the essential changes before things to escape hand.

Midlife brings exceptional wellbeing difficulties to ladies, and falling estrogen levels is only one piece of the problematic issue. Ladies need to consider other hormonal changes that happen with ageing. It's additionally critical to consider assisting with keeping cerebrum and cardiovascular wellbeing fit as a fiddle.

These are intensely impacted by way of life. Also, none of them needs to prevent you from carrying on with a happy life for a long time. You can keep yourself in the best of wellbeing, genuinely and intellectually, yet you have to stay away from some basic mix-ups.

"This is valid," Dr Alyson Pidich from The Ash Centre says. Individuals have been living longer and longer for a considerable length of time, however now they are likewise healthier. A 2016 quick survey shows that America's new most loved age is 50. The inquiry was: If you could always live healthy at a specific period, what age might you want to be? You are still youthful enough to begin once again, and savvy enough not to commit numerous errors.

Skin weakening

Ladies make some hard memories tolerating that their skin doesn't look as high, Dr Pidich says. In any case, this is an unavoidable truth, which can be taken care of. The best arrangement is something as exhausting as a keto diet and exercise. You can put certain nourishments all over for unfathomable skin, yet you additionally need to keep up a keto dietist keto diet so your skin can get all nutrients it needs to remain gleaming.

Muscle misfortune quickens

Ageing accompanies symptoms such as substantial changes in body piece, remembering an effective abatement for bulk. Fit bulk, by and large, contributes up to around 50 per cent of total body weight in youthful grown-ups, yet diminishes with age to be about 25 per cent of total body weight by age 75–80 years, as indicated by National Institutes of Health.

You lose collagen as well.

Collagen keep the body together; essentially, Dr Pidich says. It is the principle of essential protein in the space in the different connective tissues in the body. Collagen is, likewise, what gives skin immovability. Collagen creation starts typically to decrease as ladies get more seasoned, she includes. This is another motivation to eat many nourishments that are plentiful in Vitamin C – it's critical for collagen amalgamation, Dr Pidich says.

Digestion is slower

Metabolism is the procedure through which the body changes over what an individual eats into vitality. It eases back down as you lose bulk. The two are interwoven. That is the reason typical counsel specialists have for individuals who need to help their digestion is to do obstruction preparing. Additionally, individuals will, in general, be less dynamic, which can likewise destroy their metabolic procedures.

You need to do quality preparation.

Your digestion eases back down, and you lose muscle. The best way to battle these symptoms of ageing is by doing quality preparation. Further down the road, bone and bulk will result in a general reduction, adaptability begins to lessen and adjust, and readiness is now and then undermined. Studies have discovered that quality preparation can expand quality in more established grown-ups and, accordingly, empowers them to live more freely.

You, despite everything, need 7-9 hours of rest.

You may have heard that more seasoned individuals were restless, which is common, yet this is a legend, Dr Pidich says. Furthermore, it can cost you your wellbeing. "Individuals, despite everything, need to rest 7-9 hours per night. "A sleeping disorder quite often connects with menopause," she includes. This is because the ovaries steadily decline the creation of estrogen and progesterone, a rest advancing hormone, as per the National Sleep Foundation.

Treat the reason for torment, not the side effects.

Pain is usual as individuals get more established, yet it's not OK. The most significant issue is managing the wellspring of the side effects. "A great deal of torment originates from obscure provocative procedures in the body," Dr Pidich says. Is it the spine, bone, or joint pain? Back torment can be because of bulk as well as terrible stance, she includes. Ensure you do exercise to fix your position and include light loads, Dr Pidich says.

Weight gain is more straightforward.

What's more, getting in shape is a lot harder, Dr Sandra Culbertson, Chair of Women's Health at Geisinger, says. "The typical strategies don't work any longer." The reasons can shift from expanded feelings of anxiety to more slow digestion and loss of muscle. Likewise, the body holds increasingly white fat as you age. This is the caring that stores overabundance calories. You create white fat by devouring an excessive number of calories and not consuming them.

Be that as it may, most ladies overlook it.

What ladies miss the most, in Dr Culbertson's expert experience, is keeping up a stable weight. "This is because they frequently don't set aside some effort to deal with themselves." Kids, family, employment, and house tasks - these things take need, and "mothers" come last, she includes. This isn't maintainable; you need to discover and make time to put your prosperity first.

Fat gets put away in the gut region.

The abs are, shockingly, the absolute hardest muscles to tone in the body. The midriff is the first spot a great many people, especially ladies, store weight. What's more, it deteriorates as you age. It's only how the body works. A developing waistline is in ladies can be particularly valid after menopause, when muscle versus fat will, in a general, move to the stomach. This is likely because of a diminishing degree of estrogen, which seems to impact where fat is appropriated in the body.

Menopause is inescapable

This is a marked decrease in conceptive hormones, and it doesn't have extra any lady. Sooner or later, your menstrual periods stop for all time. (Some may contend this is something to be thankful for, because who needs to experience all that consistently any longer?) While menopause spurs many (once in a while uncommon) changes inside the body, practice is probably the ideal approach to help keep your physical and enthusiastic prosperity unblemished as you progress through it.

In any case, you can mitigate side effects.

Hot flashes, vaginal dryness, rest aggravations, uneasiness – these frequently accompany menopause. In any case, you don't need to persevere through the wretchedness. You can exploit hormonal substitution treatments. "A ton of ladies endure due to the myths about these treatments," Dr Culbertson says. "Some natural medications may help also."

Vaginal dryness can without much of a stretch be dealt with

"No one needs to discuss this, although it can truly affect connections," Dr Culbertson says. This can be dealt with an insignificant portion of estrogen creams. "It has a gigantic effect," she includes.

Urinary issues are regular yet not typical.

Bladder control is another issue ladies don't care to discuss. "We see a ton of urinary issue among more established ladies," Dr Culbertson says. "Individuals standardize it since it frequently happens, yet this isn't acceptable." Incontinence can run from the spilling of a couple of drops when hacking or in any event, snickering to splashing. The reason should be examined. "A simple treatment is to reinforce the pelvic floor," she includes.

You can't switch changes, yet you can back them off.

This is a practical desire, Dr Pidich says. Numerous components assume a job in whatever ageing signs a lady can understanding. Easing back them down has a great deal to do with keeping up a robust way of life. "Change doesn't occur without any forethought," she includes. This additionally applies to see receiving the rewards from a minor form of life upgrades.

Coronary illness is adversary No. 1

Coronary disease is the primary source of death for ladies in the U.S., as indicated by the CDC. The cardiovascular malady is frequently thought of as a "man's infection," however, around a similar number of ladies and men bite the dust every year accordingly. Remember that obscure manifestations, for example, the brevity of breath, weakness, expanding of the feet/lower legs/legs/mid-region, can be indications of a cardiovascular breakdown, mainly if it happens all the while. Diabetes is up there, as well.

"Serious issue in ladies I see is diabetes," Dr Pidich says. Around 15 million ladies in the nation have the condition, or about 1 in every nine grown-up ladies, as indicated by the Department of Health. Type 2 diabetes is progressively regular in grown-ups, particularly in individuals 45 and more established, have a family ancestry of diabetes, or have overweight or obesity. Contrasted and men with diabetes, ladies with diabetes, have a higher hazard for coronary illness, lower endurance rates, and more danger for visual deficiency and wretchedness.

Pay attention to keto diet insufficiency very.

Dr Pidich says she sees a shockingly high number of ladies with keto diet insufficiencies. "It's stunning to see that when everything is so promptly accessible." But what we are told is sound may not be for our bodies, she includes. That is the reason it's acceptable to test what your body can't deal with and to have an altered keto diet plan. "For instance, the GI tract doesn't retain nutrients similarly." Bonus: Weight misfortune becomes more straightforward once you treat these inadequacies, Dr Pidich includes.

Heartburn is regularly mistaken for low corrosive in the stomach.

This is one thing she sees a great deal. "Ladies come in with an analysis of heartburn when they have low corrosive in the stomach." The stomach can't separate all nourishment to retain the supplements; the extra food is then scouring against the abdomen. The disarray is effortlessly cleared with a basic test. After that, patients might be given stomach related catalysts and side effects leave, she includes.

Your body doesn't separate liquor, so no problem at all.

This may because of different reasons, including medical issues that may have created and prescriptions you're taking since some can be influenced by liquor. Since bulk is supplanted by fat tissue as individuals get more established, drinking a similar sum as when they were more youthful outcomes in a higher blood liquor fixation. The liquor remains longer in your stream, increment its danger of harm. Bloodstream to it is likewise diminished.

The typical weight doesn't mean a sound individual.

BMI doesn't give you a sensible proportion of how rational you are, Dr Pidich says. It's imperative to consider your tallness and weight, yet the level of fat and muscle in your body. However, look different. (Muscle is a lot littler.) Two individuals may have similar BMI regardless of whether one of them seems a lot more slender than the other.

Auspicious screening can spare your life.

Modern screening makes it conceivable to recognize existing tumours at the beginning period when treatment is beneficial. However, 33% of patients kick the bucket, making the disease of the internal organ the following driving reason for malignant growth passings in ladies in the U.S., as indicated by the Center for Menstrual Disorders. Mammograms, as well, Dr Culbertson, include.

Get your skin looked at

Skin malignancy increments as individuals get more seasoned. A full skin test by a dermatologist or clinical expert is perhaps the best methodologies for distinguishing it. This can spare your life. When a disease has advanced and spread, it is increasingly hard to treat with a lot of more mediocre and results. An individual with healthy skin, with no particular issues and no family ancestry of melanoma or other skin tumours, ought to experience such a test once per year.

Eating less won't bring about weight reduction.

Hormonal changes are a significant factor in not having the option to shed pounds as quickly, Dr Pidich says. Keto diet inadequacies contribute too because the body feels like it's destitute, she includes. Be that as it may, eating less doesn't work, particularly after 50. "Starving the body doesn't rise to weight reduction." You need to do it in a way the body can endure – increment bulk, eat healthy nourishment a couple of times each day, and accomplish progressively high-impact exercises.

Try not to succumb to popular fashion keto diets.

Probably the enormous misstep individuals can make to look to FAD keto diets to get thinner, particularly when there's not long to go until the get-away time this season, Yvonne Sanders of Slimming World, who shed 63 pounds herself. These plans are frequently excessively prohibitive. Your body needs all the supplements; it can find a proper pace thickness and bulk. You can wind up being malnourished.

Stress is a quiet executioner.

It can happen at any age. However, it has a higher effect on ladies more than 50. "We can see in the blood's work," she includes. Thyroid organs and adrenal capacity, among different organs, are influenced. Stress takes a higher physical cost when you're more seasoned, she includes. Your body is ageing, and your heart wellness and lung limit decrease. Stress hormones in the cerebrum can likewise add to transient memory issues that are random to dementia, as per Harvard Medical School.

Cerebral pains might be an indication of a significant issue.

Cerebral pains can be a significant issue as you get more seasoned, Dr Pidich says. Most are anything but difficult to fix since they are because of a lack of hydration. However, cerebral pains can likewise mean aneurysm or stroke she includes. "An aneurysm has, for the most part, been there for a short time, just not analyzed. As you get more established, the veins debilitate, collagen separates, and the divider around the aneurysm separate, and it can crack."

Stomach torment should be explored.

Stomach torment is regular among more established patients. However, it should be looked at, mainly if it's extreme or going on for a couple of days. It can mean stomach aortic aneurysm crack or lacking bloodstream to the small digestive system.

The therapeutic methodology is just transitory.

"Possibly do a system on the off chance that you will change your keto diet," Dr Pidich says. If you experience a corrective system, you may look fantastic, yet the skin will return to what it was on the off chance that you don't make the fundamental way of life transforms, she includes. The greatest kindness you can accomplish for your skin is to take care of its nutritious nourishment. Bloodstream supplies it with what it needs to gleam. On the off chance that you, despite everything, eat poorly, the skin won't get the reliable supplements it needs and will get dry and wrinkled.

Ovarian malignant growth is dealt with most successfully when distinguished early

66% of diseases are believed to be because of arbitrary transformations, and most ovarian malignancies are in that class, as per Dr John P. Micha, organizer of the Nancy Yeary Women's Cancer Research Foundation. They are a result of the various cell divisions the bodies experience day by day. The ovarian disease is frequently analyzed in its propelled stages because there are no robust screening strategies, and ladies regularly accept that manifestations like extreme swelling, stomach torment, and draining are just identified with minor issues.

Remaining truly dynamic is vital.

On the chance that there are one thing ladies more than 50 ought to do consistently, it would be exercise or some type of physical activity, Dr Culbertson says. Having an inactive existence is staggeringly undesirable; "a great many people have no clue," she includes. A great many people go through about a large portion of the day sitting. The body isn't prepared to be in one situation for a long time. "You must find a good pace."

So is extending

Adaptability is one of the most significant objectives of wellness. It's similarly as vital as being reliable and fit. The capacity to handily move around is urgent for forestalling wounds, falls and back torment, expanding blood supply and supplements to the muscles, diminishing irritation, and improving stance. Muscle tissues and tendons turn out to be less flexible with time – only one more motivation to require some investment and stretch.

You can, in any case, drink – with some restraint.

You have presumably known about the most recent examination on liquor's impact on an individual's wellbeing. The reality, as per it, is that no measure of alcohol is sheltered. Specialists, in any case, are not in a race to sound the caution. On the off chance that you separate the numbers and indeed read into how they did the investigation, as The New York Times did, you'll see that there is no compelling reason to blow a gasket. "Everything with some restraint," Dr Pidich says.

Try not to overlook sore calves.

It might be something beyond a muscle strain; it could be deep vein thrombosis (DVT), blood coagulation in your veins. It tends to be risky whenever left untreated. Blood clusters in your veins can loosen up, travel through your circulatory system and cabin in your lungs, blocking bloodstream (aspiratory embolism). Red or stained skin on the leg is another side effect.

Hearing misfortune is conceivable.

While most hearing misfortune happens in the old, ladies in their middle age can encounter it, as well. Clamours become quieted when the hair cells in your internal ear are harmed or kick the bucket. They don't develop back, so the misfortune is changeless. Presentation to boisterous commotions, family ancestry, smoking, diabetes, and chemotherapy medications can likewise assume a job in hearing trouble.

You likely need multivitamins and enhancements.

You should take supplements not to advance weight, yet instead to detoxify the body and give it a supplement that it is insufficient. It is Dr Daryl Gioffre, big-name keto dietist and creator of getting OFF YOUR ACID, says. "For instance, if a plant shrinks, you give it water since it needs water, and our bodies are the same." There are a couple of enhancements that we are, for the most part, insufficient in, even kids, yet you, despite everything, need to run these by your human services professional, he includes.

Visit an eye specialist once every year.

Your vision starts to fall apart after you hit 40. Your eyes lose flexibility, and they become unfit to centre. A white ring or band around the iris could be a sign of elevated cholesterol. In more established grown-ups, the ring is brought about by fat and cholesterol stores. It is typical; however, in individuals more youthful than 60, it could show elevated cholesterol and greater danger of coronary episode and stroke.

You need increasingly solid fats.

Try not to be apprehensive from "fats." Keto dietary fats are essential to give your body vitality and to help cell development, as indicated by the American Heart Association. They help secure your organs, the body assimilates a few supplements and produces significant hormones. Fish, nuts and seeds, are fantastic wellsprings of polyunsaturated and monounsaturated unsaturated fats.

Ladies with little calves might be bound to have a stroke.

A recent report has proposed that ladies whose calves are 13 inches or less have a more prominent possibility of creating carotid plaque, a condition where plaque develops inside the corridors. This can prompt a stroke. Paying attention to the size of your calves, heart maladies are anything but difficult to forestall with a solid keto diet and a consistent exercise plan.

Hair diminishing and blurring are conceivable.

The shade cells in your hair follicles will begin to die, and the strands won't have the option to keep up as much melanin. This is the reason hair turns dim, silver, or white. As ladies get more seasoned, their estrogen levels decay. Adequate degrees of estrogen represent a thick head of hair, so without quite a bit of it, strands can turn out to be meagre, dry, weak, or drop out by and large.

Deal with your gut

A developing group of research shows that the state of the stomach related framework assumes a colossal job in one's general wellbeing. Scientists are finding a reliable connection between stomach related wellbeing and the cerebrum. By impacting the parity and kinds of microbes present, it considers showing that it might be conceivable to bring down pressure, influence discernment/mind procedures and mind-set. Would you be able to do to upgrade your stomach related wellbeing? Certain nourishments like yoghurt, sauerkraut, a fermented tea, and coconut Keifer can help keep up the "great" microorganisms expected to keep your gut running smoothly.

Don't try too hard with the hot showers.

Long hot showers are pleasant and unwinding, yet in all actuality, they are damaging your skin. The warmth from the water evacuates your skin's oil hindrance, which causes irritated, dry, and wrinkling skin. Research has demonstrated that chilly showers can help decrease the presence of skin break out.

Try not to disregard the smell of your pee.

You shouldn't have the option to recognize an odour after you pee. Pee that contains a great deal of water and not many waste items has practically no smell. "On the chance that pee turns out to be profoundly focused, your pee may have a robust alkali smell. Malodorous pee can indicate uncontrolled diabetes, a metabolic issue, UTI, and bladder aggravation.

There is no wonder solution for cellulite.

Tragic, however evident. What's more, the exhausting answer is that weight reduction and exercise can help improve the presence of cellulite. Supplanting fat with a tissue can likewise make cellulite less observable, as indicated by the American Academy of Dermatology. Various treatments treat cellulite, yet results differ, and, much of the time, rehashed meetings are required.

Walk heel-to-toe

How you walk is significant for which muscles in your body are working and for generally vitality effectiveness. Strolling heel to toe is, for people, the most proficient way. It takes almost twice as much vitality to walk on your toes than it does to arrive on your heel. Notwithstanding that, on the off chance that you walk in a toes-to-heels way, at that point, you're lessening the sum your Achilles ligament extends, and your soleus muscles (under the knee to the heel) don't fill in to such an extent.

Terrible breath can be a sign of a genuine medical problem.

Salivation acts like a cleaning specialist; it disposes of appalling microbes in your mouth. At the point when spit creation is diminished, now and then because of lack of hydration, you get a terrible breath. Be that as it may, the reasons can be significantly more genuine. You may have contamination (this occurs typically after tooth evacuation), or your teeth might be rotting. A few malignant growths, and conditions, for example, metabolic scatters, can cause an unmistakable breath scent because of synthetic substances they produce.

Get tried for nourishment bigotries.

Undiscovered nourishment bigotries can be the motivation behind why you're continuously drained, regardless of whether you get enough rest. Any nourishment – irrespective of whether dairy, grains or even chocolate – that an individual is adversely affected by causes much additional weight on the body. Usually, the body's safe framework will attempt to battle it, bringing about irritation that can extend from joint agony to cerebral pains to a growth in the small digestive tract.

Plunk down to eat

A recent report that included grown-up ladies presumed that the average individual would devour less nourishment and fewer calories when plunking down to eat, Dr Gioffre says. "The point when you take a look at this from a good judgment viewpoint, individuals who stand when they eat, are normally doing so because they are focused or in a rush, and generally a mix of the two." When you are sincerely focused on, your body will deliver less hydrochloric corrosive (HCL), which is vital for the legitimate processing of nourishment. The point when you plunk down to eat, you're bound to eat gradually.

You ought to get a screen for wretchedness.

Studies in family practice and general medication facilities demonstrate that 11 to 33 per cent of more established patients have probably a few side effects of sorrow, as indicated by AAFP. Misery at a later stage in life is generally mistaken for conceivable reactions of different ailments and drugs individuals take for them.

Week of the keto diet meal plan

Monday

Scrambled eggs (breakfast)

Spread in addition to eggs, rises to the ideal keto breakfast. Start your day away directly with our particularly productive and fulfilling form of this morning meal great. We are prepared in minutes!

Ingredients

- 1 oz. spread
- Two eggs
- salt and pepper

Instructions

Break the eggs into a little bowl and utilize a fork to whisk them together with some salt and pepper.

Dissolve the spread in a non-stick skillet over medium warmth. Watch the range cautiously shouldn't turn dark coloured!

Empty the eggs into the skillet and mix for 1 2 minutes, until they are smooth and cooked how you like them. Recollect that the eggs will at present be cooking much after you've put them on your plate.

Keto Asian hamburger salad (lunch)

Gingery and flavorful with a marginally hot kick. Generous red meat with velvety sesame goodness. All that, keto, and a reviving plate of mixed greens for sure? Do you see where we're going with this? Meet your most up to date most loved nourishment in a bowl!

Ingredients

- Sesame mayonnaise
- ¾ cup mayonnaise
- 1 tsp sesame oil
- ½ tbsp lime juice
- salt and pepper

Meat

- 1 tbsp olive oil
- 1 tbsp fish sauce
- 1 tbsp ground new ginger
- 1 tsp stew pieces
- 2/3 lb ribeye steaks
- The plate of mixed greens
- 3 oz. cherry tomatoes
- 2 oz. cucumber
- 3 oz. lettuce
- ½ red onion
- new cilantro
- 1 tsp sesame seeds
- Two scallions

Instructions

Set up the sesame mayonnaise by blending mayo in with the sesame oil and lime juice. Season with salt and pepper. Put in a safe spot.

Blend all ingredients for the hamburger marinade and fill a plastic sack. Include the hamburger and marinate for 15 minutes or more at room temperature.

Cleave all vegetables for the serving of mixed greens, except the scallions, into reduced down pieces—the separation between two plates.

Warmth a medium grill over medium heat. Add sesame seeds to the dry skillet, and toast them for two or three minutes, or until they're softly seared and fragrant. Put in a safe spot.

Pat the meat dry on the two sides with paper towels. On high warmth, burn for a moment or two on each side, and afterwards diminish warmth to medium-low, cooking until hamburger is medium, and eventually move to a cutting board.

Fry the scallions for a moment in a similar dish.

Cut the meat, over the grain, into thin cuts—Spot meat and scallions on the vegetables.

Top with broiled sesame seeds and present with a spot of sesame mayonnaise as an afterthought.

Keto pesto chicken dish with feta cheddar and olives (dinner)

Mediterranean whizzes feta cheddar, olives, and pesto join right now, to-make keto chicken dish. In the case of utilizing low-carb, locally acquired, or your home-made pesto, give it a go. Your taste buds and your family will much be obliged!

Ingredients

- 1½ lbs boneless chicken thighs or chicken bosoms
- salt and pepper
- 2 tbsp margarine or coconut oil
- 5 tbsp red pesto or green pesto
- 1¼ cups substantial whipping cream
- 3 oz. pitted olives
- 5 oz. feta cheddar, diced
- One garlic clove, finely cleaved

For serving

- 5 oz. verdant greens
- 4 tbsp olive oil
- ocean salt and ground dark pepper

Instructions

Heat the grill to 400°F.

Cut the chicken into reduced down pieces—season with salt and pepper.

Add margarine or oil to a considerable skillet and fry the chicken pieces in bunches on medium-high warmth until brilliant darker.

Utilizing locally acquired low-carb red or green pesto, or making your own, blend pesto and overwhelming cream in a bowl.

Spot the singed chicken types in a heating hand out with olives, feta cheddar, and garlic. Include the pesto/cream blend.

Prepare in the stove for 20-30 minutes, until the dish turns bubbly and light dark coloured around the edges.

Tuesday

Keto cheddar roll-ups (breakfast)

Gracious, yes. This is the quickest, easiest, most keto-lip-smacking formula known to humankind. It's difficult to oppose its exquisite goodness!

Ingredients

•   8 oz. cheddar or provolone cheddar or Edam cheddar, in cuts

•   2 oz. margarine

Instructions

Spot the cheddar cuts on a large cutting board.

Cut margarine with a cheddar slicer or cut truly slender pieces with a blade.

Spread each cheddar cut with flatter and roll. Fill in as a bite.

Keto Caprice omelette (lunch)

Delicate mozzarella, ready tomatoes, and new basil, yes, please! In an egg, surprisingly better! This super-simple, keto dish works for breakfast, lunch or dinner, and makes sure to be another fave. So get out your grill Italy, here we come!

Ingredients

•   Six eggs

•   salt and pepper

•   1 tbsp hacked new basil or dried basil

•   2 tbsp olive oil

•   3 oz. cherry tomatoes cut in equal parts or plants cut in cuts

•   5 oz. fresh mozzarella cheddar, diced or cut

Instructions

Break the eggs into a blending bowl, add salt and dark pepper precisely as you would prefer.

Whisk well with a fork until completely consolidated. Include basil and mix.

Warmth oil in a huge skillet. Fry the tomatoes for a couple of moments.

Pour the egg player on the tomatoes. Hold up until the hitter is marginally firm before including the mozzarella cheddar.

Lower the warmth and let the omelette set. Serve immediately and appreciate it!

Keto meat pie (dinner)

Keep everybody content with this fantastic; cheddar bested keto showstopper. Meat pie might be a little old fashioned. However, it's an excellent opportunity to rediscover its scrumptiousness. Any cook can get rave surveys with this simple-to-follow formula.

Ingredients

Pie outside

- ¾ cup almond flour
- 4 tbsp sesame seeds
- 4 tbsp coconut flour
- 1 tbsp ground psyllium husk powder
- 1 tsp preparing powder
- One squeeze salt
- 3 tbsp olive oil or coconut oil, dissolved
- One egg
- 4 tbsp water

Besting

- 8 oz. curds
- 7 oz. destroyed cheddar

Filling

- ½ yellow onion, finely hacked
- One garlic clove, finely hacked
- 2 tbsp spread or olive oil
- 1¼ lbs ground meat or ground sheep
- 1 tbsp dried oregano/basil
- salt and pinch of pepper
- 4 tbsp tomato glue or ajvar relish
- ½ cup of water

Instructions

Heat the stove to 350°F.

Fry onion and garlic in spread or olive oil over medium warmth for a couple of moments until onion is delicate. Include ground meat and continue broiling. Include oregano or basil—salt and pepper to taste.

Include tomato glue or ajvar relish. Include water. Lower the warmth and let stew for at any rate 20 minutes. While the meat stews, make the mixture for the hull.

Blend all the covering ingredients in a nourishment processor for a couple of moments until the batter transforms into a ball. On the chance that you don't have a nourishment processor, you can blend by hand with a fork.

Spot a round bit of material paper in an all-around lubed springform container or deep-dish pie skillet 9-10 inches (23-25 cm) in width to make it simpler to evacuate the pie's set. Spread the batter in the box and up at the edges. Utilize a spatula or very much lubed fingers. When the covering is moulded to the skillet, prick the base of the outside layer with a fork.

Pre-prepare the covering for 10-15 minutes. Expel from the stove and spot the meat in the coating: blend curds and destroyed cheddar together, and layer on the pie.

Prepare on the lower rack for 30-40 minutes or until the pie has turned a brilliant shading.

Wednesday
Keto frittata with new spinach (breakfast)
This stunning dish looks past high, yet is incredibly easy to make! Spinach, eggs, sausage or bacon, and veggies mysteriously join into a heavenly gala for the eyes and the belly. It's keto gold!
Ingredients
- 5 oz. diced bacon or chorizo
- 2 tbsp spread
- 8 oz. new spinach
- Eight eggs
- 1 cup overwhelming whipping cream
- 5 oz. destroyed cheddar
- salt and pepper

Instructions
Heat the stove to 350°F. Oil a 9x9 preparing dish or individual ramekins.

Fry the bacon in a spread on medium warmth until fresh. Include the spinach and mix until withered. Expel the dish from the heat and put it in a safe spot.

Whisk the eggs and cream together and fill the heating dish or in ramekins.

Include the bacon, spinach, and cheddar on top and spot in the stove. Heat for 25 30 minutes or until set in the centre and brilliant darker on top.

Keto no-noodle chicken soup (lunch)

Made with recuperating bone stock, this keto chicken no-noodle soup with sound cabbage is warm and soothing when it's cold outside when you're battling a cold, or you simply ache for a healthy soup!

Ingredients

- 4 oz. margarine
- 2 tbsp dried minced onion
- Two celery stalks, slashed
- 6 oz. mushrooms, cut
- Two minced garlic cloves
- 8 cups of chicken juices
- One medium measured carrot, cut
- 2 tsp dried parsley
- 1 tsp salt
- ¼ tsp ground dark pepper
- 1½ rotisserie chicken, destroyed
- 5 oz. green cabbage, cut into strips

Instructions

Soften the margarine in an enormous pot, over medium warmth.

Include dried onion, slashed celery, cut mushrooms and garlic into the pot and cook for 3-4 minutes.

Include juices, cut carrot, parsley, salt, and pepper. Stew until vegetables are delicate.

Include cooked chicken and cabbage. Stew for an extra 8-12 minutes until the cabbage "noodles" is delicate.

Keto pasta carbonara (dinner)

Zucchini noodles or zoodles are something beyond an "elective" to standard pasta. They're a culinary treat! With all the velvety surfaces and fresh bacon mash of the Italian exemplary, this snappy and fulfilling keto formula hits quite a few notes.

Ingredients

- 1¼ cups substantial whipping cream
- 1 tbsp margarine
- 10 oz. bacon
- ¼ cup of mayonnaise
- salt pinch and pepper
- 2 lbs zucchini
- Four egg yolks
- 3 oz. ground parmesan cheddar, some more for serving

Instructions

Empty the substantial cream into a sauce skillet, and heat it to the point of boiling over medium-high warmth. Lower the warmth to medium-low, and let bubble for a couple of moments until diminished by a fourth.

In a large skillet, liquefy the spread over medium warmth. Add bacon to the dish, fricasseeing until fresh. Put bacon in a safe spot. Keep the fat warm in the recipe, on the lowest setting.

Whisk the mayonnaise into the substantial cream. Salt and a pinch of pepper for taste, and cook until mayonnaise is warmed and cooked adequately. Decrease temperature to low, blending at times.

Make zucchini spirals with a spiralizer or through potato peeler.

Spot zoodles in a microwave-safe bowl, and microwave on high for 3-5 minutes, until warmed through, yet have a new, firm surface. On the chance that you would prefer not to microwave, you can heat the zoodles in boiling water for 30 seconds.

In a different bowl, consolidate the egg yolks, diced bacon, and parmesan cheddar.

Include the bacon fat and the warm cream sauce to the zoodles, hurling together until zoodles are covered. Guarantee that this blend is somewhat mild, and afterwards include the egg-bacon-parmesan cheddar blend to the zoodles, throwing all along (the egg blend will scramble if too warm when consolidating).

The separation between four plates. Top with a liberal measure of newly ground parmesan.

Thursday

Without dairy keto latte (breakfast)

Latte? Indeed, it would be ideal if you This sans dairy enchant is the ideal in a hurried breakfast. Five minutes to blend it up, and you're finished. Voila! It's a keto enchantment!

Ingredients

- Two eggs
- 2 tbsp coconut oil
- 1½ cups bubbling water
- One squeeze vanilla concentrate
- 1 tsp pumpkin pie zest or ground ginger

Instructions

Mix all ingredients in a blender. You should be speedy, so the eggs don't cook in the bubbling water! Drink right away.

Tip!

In case you're longing for hot cocoa, or simply need a plain latte, supplant the flavours with one tablespoon of cocoa or moment espresso. Presto!

Keto avocado, bacon and goat-cheddar salad (lunch)

Are you searching for a supervisor plate of mixed greens? Longing for velvety avocados and goat cheddar with the smash of nuts? Goodness, man. Do we have a formula for you! Arrange this for a helping quick lunch or dinner.

Ingredients

- 8 oz. goat cheddar
- 8 oz. bacon
- Two avocados
- 4 oz. arugula lettuce

- 4 oz. pecans

Dressing

- 1 tbsp lemon, the juice
- ½ cup mayonnaise
- ½ cup olive oil
- 2 tbsp overwhelming whipping cream
- salt and pepper

Instructions

Heat the stove to 200°C and place the material paper in a heating dish.

Cut the goat cheddar into round half-inch (~1 cm) cuts and spot in the preparing dish. Heat on upper rack until brilliant.

Fry the bacon in a container until fresh.

Cut the avocado into pieces and put on the arugula. Include the singed bacon and goat cheddar. Sprinkle nuts on top.

Utilizing a submersion blender, make the dressing with the lemon juice, mayonnaise, olive oil, and cream—season with salt and pepper to taste.

Tip!

Are you searching for somewhat more antipatent? While this dressing is delectable all alone, don't hesitate to add your preferred herbs to make it much progressively powerful. Fresh parsley, dill, or thyme, will balance the dressing unbelievably well.

Keto pizza (dinner)

Pizza, meet keto. It's a straightforward interpretation of how to get your pizza fix without the carbs. It's all that you need regardless of whether it is a straightforward pepperoni, cheddar, and tomato-sauce rendition, or a stacked party. Make it your own.

Ingredients

- Four eggs
- 6 oz. destroyed cheddar, ideally mozzarella or provolone
- Besting
- 3 tbsp unsweetened tomato sauce
- 1 tsp dried oregano
- 5 oz. destroyed cheddar

- • 1½ oz. pepperoni
- • olives (discretionary)

For serving

- • 2 oz. verdant greens
- • 4 tbsp olive oil
- • ocean salt and ground dark pepper

Instructions

Heat the stove to 400°F.

Start by making the hull. Split eggs into a and include cheddar. Give it a decent mix to join.

Use a spatula to spread it hitter against a heating sheet fixed with material paper. You can shape two circles or simply make one huge rectangular pizza. Prepare in the grill for 15 minutes until the pizza outside layer turns brilliant. Expel and let cool for a moment or two.

Increment the broiler temperature to 450°F (225°C).

Spread tomato sauce on the covering and sprinkle oregano on top. Top with cheddar and put some of the pepperoni or olives on it.

Heat for another 5-10 min until pizza has turned a brilliant darker shading.

Present with a crisp palate of mixed greens as an afterthought.

Friday

Keto mushroom omelette (breakfast)

Are you searching for a brisk and straightforward approach to begin your day? This generous omelette is excessively solid, and just takes a couple of moments to make! Fresh mushrooms make a tasty filling. Appreciate this keto meal whenever breakfast, lunch, or dinner!

Ingredients

- • Three eggs
- • 1 oz. spread, for broiling
- • 1 oz. cheddar
- • ¼ yellow onion, hacked
- • Four huge mushrooms, cut
- • salt and pepper

Instructions

Break the eggs into a blending bowl in with a spot of salt and pepper. Whisk the eggs with a fork until smooth and foamy.

Soften the spread in a skillet, over medium warmth. Add the mushrooms and onion to the dish, blending until delicate, and afterwards pour in the egg blend, encompassing the veggies.

At the point when the omelette starts to cook and get firm, yet at the same time has a little crude egg on top, sprinkle cheddar over the egg.

Utilizing a spatula, cautiously ease around the edges of the omelette, and afterwards overlap it over into equal parts. At the point when it begins to turn brilliant dark coloured underneath, expel the dish from the warmth and slide the omelette on to a plate.

Keto smoked salmon plate (lunch)

Genuine nourishment on a plate. Salmon. Spinach. Mayo and lime.

Ingredients

- ¾ lb smoked salmon
- 1 cup mayonnaise
- 2 oz. infant spinach
- 1 tbsp olive oil
- ½ lime (discretionary)
- salt and pinch of black pepper

Instructions

Put salmon and spinach, a wedge of lime and a generous touch of mayonnaise on a plate.

Sprinkle olive oil over the spinach and season with salt and pepper.

Tip!

Swap out the salmon for any greasy fish you appreciate. (Mackerel, herring, sardines, and anchovies are, for the most part, excellent alternatives.) You can likewise change the greens attempt destroyed cabbage or hot arugula.

Keto tortilla with ground hamburger and salsa (dinner)

Treat yourself to a beautiful meat-and-cheddar filled tortilla. With your custom made keto bread and flavour blend, this Mexican most loved won't just be energizing, yet additionally heavenly!

Ingredients

Low-carb tortillas

- Two eggs

- Two egg whites
- 5 oz. cream cheddar, relaxed
- ½ tsp salt
- 1½ tsp ground psyllium husk powder
- 1 tbsp coconut flour

Filling
- 2 tbsp olive oil
- 1 lb ground hamburger or ground sheep, at room temperature
- 2 tbsp Tex-Mex flavouring
- ½ cup of water
- salt and pepper

Salsa
- Two avocados, diced
- One tomato, diced
- 2 tbsp lime juice
- 1 tbsp olive oil
- ½ cup crisp cilantro, cleaved
- salt and pepper

For serving
- 6 oz. destroyed Mexican cheddar
- 3 oz. destroyed lettuce

Low-carb tortillas

Heat the grill/oven to 400°F.

Utilizing an electric blender with the whisk connection, whisk the eggs and egg whites until feathery, ideally for a couple of moments. In a different enormous bowl, beat the cream cheddar until smooth. Add the eggs to the cream cheddar, and speed until the eggs and cream cheddar structure a steady player.

Blend salt, psyllium husk, and coconut flour in a little bowl. Include the flour blend each spoon in turn into the player and keep on whisking some more. Let the hitter sit for a couple of moments or until the player is thick, similar to an American flapjack player. How quickly the player will grow relies upon the brand of psyllium husk. Some experimentation may be required.

Bring out two preparing sheets and spot material paper on each. Utilizing a spatula, spread the hitter daintily (close to ¼ inch thick) into 4 6 circles or 2 square shapes.

Prepare on the upper rack for around 5 minutes or more, until the tortilla turns somewhat dark-coloured around the edges. Cautiously check the base side with the goal that it doesn't consume.

Filling

Spot an enormous grill over medium-high warmth and warmth up the oil. Include the ground hamburger and fry until cooked.

Include the tex-mex flavouring and water and mix. Let stew until the vast majority of the water is no more. Taste to check whether it needs extra flavour.

Saturday

Keto heated bacon omelette (breakfast)

Bacon, to say the least, for breakfast, lunch, or dinner. The spinach mixes it up. The eggs hold everything together. Be that as it may, bacon rules. Keto life is acceptable.

Ingredients

- Four eggs
- 5 oz. bacon cut in 3D squares
- 3 oz. spread
- 2 oz. new spinach
- 1 tbsp finely hacked crisp chives (discretionary)
- salt and pepper

Instructions

Heat the stove to 400°F. Oil an individual serving-sized heating dish with the spread.

Fry bacon and spinach in the rest of the spread.

Whisk the eggs until foamy. Blend in the spinach and bacon, including the fat left from fricasseeing.

Include some finely cleaved chives—season to taste with salt and pepper.

Empty the egg blend into prepared dish(es) and heat for 20 minutes or until set and brilliant dark-coloured.

Let cool for a couple of moments and serve.

Tip!

If you love cheddar, you should blend in some ground cheddar or sprinkle parmesan on top before heating. Sautéed onions are another yummy conceivable expansion.

Keto quesadillas (lunch)

Concoct this brisk and simple scrumptiousness ASAP. Wanton. Mushy. Furthermore, formally keto! Scrumptious and enough to make you resemble a prominent name gourmet specialist. Serve them up as is or decked-out with sharp cream, guacamole, and salsa.

Ingredients

Low-carb tortillas

- Two eggs
- Two egg whites
- 6 oz. cream cheddar
- ½ tsp salt
- 1½ tsp ground psyllium husk powder
- 1 tbsp coconut flour

Filling

- 1 tbsp olive oil or spread, for searing
- 5 oz. Mexican cheddar or any hard cheddar of your loving
- 1 oz. infant spinach

Instructions

Tortillas

Heat the grill to 400°F.

Utilizing an electric blender, beat eggs and egg whites together until fleecy. Add cream cheddar and keep on beating until the player is smooth.

In a bowl, join salt, psyllium husk, and coconut flour. Blend well.

Include the flour blend into the player while beating. At the point when joined, let the hitter sit for a couple of moments. It ought to be thick, similar to flapjack hitter. Your image of psyllium husk powder influences this progression is understanding. If it doesn't thicken enough, include some more.

Spot material paper on a preparing sheet. Utilize a spatula to spread the hitter over the material paper into a significant square shape. On the off chance that you need round tortillas, you can sear them in a skillet like hotcakes.

Heat on the upper rack for around 5 10 minutes, until the tortilla turns dark coloured around the edges. Watch out for the stove. Don't let these delectable manifestations consume on the base!

Cut the large tortilla into smaller pieces (6 pieces for each preparing sheet).

Quesadillas

Warmth oil or spread in a little, non-stick skillet over medium warmth.

Put a tortilla in the skillet and sprinkle with cheddar, spinach, and with some more cheddar. Top with another tortilla.

Fry every quesadilla for about a moment on each side. You'll know it's done when the cheddar liquefies.

Keto Asian cabbage mix fry (dinner)

This beautiful keto pan-fried food isn't just simple to make yet, besides, incredibly delicious. This crunchy pleasure may get one of your most loved go-to plans. Think about awkward it today around the evening time!

Ingredients

- 1½ lbs green cabbage
- 4 oz. spread, partitioned
- 1 tsp salt
- 1 tsp onion powder
- ¼ tsp ground dark pepper
- 1 tbsp white wine vinegar
- Two garlic cloves, minced
- 1 tsp stew pieces
- 1 tbsp new ginger, finely cleaved or ground
- 1¼ lbs ground meat
- Three scallions, hacked in 1/2-inch cuts
- 1 tbsp sesame oil
- Wasabi mayonnaise
- 1 cup mayonnaise
- ½ tbsp wasabi glue

Instructions

Shred the cabbage finely utilizing a sharp blade or a nourishment processor.

Fry the cabbage in half of the spread in a considerable broiling or wok dish on medium-high warmth. It takes some time to relax; however, don't let it turn darker.

Include flavours and vinegar. Mix and fry for a few minutes more. Put the cabbage in a bowl.

Soften the remainder of the margarine in a similar skillet. Include garlic, stew chips, and ginger. Sauté for a couple of moments.

Include ground meat and darker until the beef is altogether cooked, and the vast majority of the juices have dissipated. Lower the warmth a bit.

Add scallions and cabbage to the meat. Mix until everything is hot—salt and pepper to taste. Sprinkle with sesame oil before serving.

Combine the wasabi mayonnaise by beginning with a modest quantity of wasabi and including more until the flavour is perfect. Serve the sautéed food warm with a spot of wasabi mayonnaise on top.

Sunday

Keto hotcakes with berries and whipped cream(breakfast)

Attempt these staggering keto curds hotcakes, and you'll never return to customary pancakes! Our berry beating gives them the perfect measure of sweetness, and the children will cherish them!

Ingredients

- Hotcakes
- Four eggs
- 7 oz. curds
- 1 tbsp ground psyllium husk powder
- 2 oz. margarine or coconut oil
- Garnishes
- 2 oz. crisp raspberries or new blueberries or new strawberries
- 1 cup substantial whipping cream

Instructions

Include eggs, curds, and psyllium husk to a medium-size bowl and combine. Let sit for 5-10 minutes.

Warmth up margarine or oil in a non-stick skillet. Fry the hotcakes on medium-low heat for 3 4 minutes on each side. Try not to make them too enormous, or they will be challenging to flip.

Add cream to a different bowl and whip until delicate pinnacles structure.

Serve the flapjacks with your preferred whipped cream and berries.

Italian keto plate (lunch)

Genuine nourishment on a plate. Prosciutto. Mozzarella. Tomatoes and olives.

Ingredients

7 oz. new mozzarella cheddar

7 oz. prosciutto, cut

Two tomatoes

1/3 cup olive oil

Ten green olives

salt and pepper

Instructions

Put tomatoes, prosciutto, cheddar, and olives on a plate. Present with olive oil and season with salt and pepper to taste.

Tip!

Swap out the prosciutto for another greasy Italian shop meat. Soppressata, coppa, or spot ring a bell. What's your top pick?

Pork hacks with green beans and garlic butter (dinner)

Succulent pork slashes. Crunchy green beans. Garlic spread. Well, that is the thing that we call a one-skillet wonder. What's more, it's keto tastefulness at its best.

Ingredients

- Garlic spread
- 5 oz. spread, at room temperature
- ½ tbsp garlic powder
- 1 tbsp dried parsley
- 1 tbsp lemon juice
- salt and pepper
- Pork hacks
- Four pork hacks
- 2 oz. spread, for singing
- 1 lb new green beans

- Salt also, pepper

Instructions

Blend spread, garlic, parsley, and lemon juice. Season with salt and pepper to taste. Put in a safe spot.

Make some little cuts in the fat encompassing the cleaves to assist them with a remaining level when searing season with salt and pepper.

In a large grill, liquefy the margarine over medium-high warmth. Include the cleaves and fry for around 5 minutes on each side or until brilliant dark coloured and altogether cooked through.

Expel the hacks from the dish and keep warm.

Utilize a similar skillet and include the beans—salt and pepper to taste. Cook over medium-high warmth until the seeds have an energetic shading and are marginally mollified yet, at the same time, a piece crunchy.

Serve the pork cleaves and beans together with a touch of garlic spread liquefying on top.

Tip!

Canned or solidified green beans may not be very as crunchy, yet at the same time taste extraordinary and convey pure supplements directly from your cooler or washroom.

Chapter 6: Keto Recipes

Keto Buns
Planning Time: 10 minutes Cook
Time: 10 minutes Total
Time: 20 minutes
Servings: 3
Calories: 708kcal
Fixings
- Blue Cheese Burgers
- 1-pound American Kobe Beef or grass bolstered 16 oz/g
- One tablespoon Worcestershire sauce
- One tablespoon Mc Cornick Montreal Steak Seasoning
- 4 ounces disintegrated blue cheddar
- Flame-broiled Marinated Portobello Mushrooms
- Three medium portobello mushrooms
- 4 ounces onion cut into rings
- 1/4 cup low carb Italian Salad Dressing
- Compound Butter (discretionary)
- 1 oz stick spread, delicate
- 2 ounces disintegrated blue cheddar
- One tablespoon minced parsley
- Two teaspoons minced shallot

Directions
Compound Butter: Mince the parsley and shallot. Put the range in a little bowl. Mix or squash with a fork until smooth. Mix in the disintegrated blue cheddar, shallot, and parsley until consolidated. Scoop the compound spread onto a bit of waxed paper, focusing it the long way down the centre of the article. Fold into a log, bend the closures, and store at a low temperature.

Mushrooms and Onions: Cut the onion into 1/4 - 1/3-inch rings. With a medium estimated spoon, scratch out the gills from the mushrooms. Empty the serving of mixed greens dressing into a bowl and dunk the truffles into the dressing, appropriating the dressing on all surfaces. Coat the onions with the remainder of the dressing. Flame broil the Portobellos on the barbecue, gill side down first, and flip to get done with cooking. Cook the onions to burn them a piece. Spot the mushrooms and onions on a platter and tent with foil to keep warm.

Blue Cheese Burgers: Break up the ground hamburger. If it separates into excessively modest pieces, include two tablespoons of oil. Additionally, add the oil on the off chance that you are utilizing grass-nourished meat since that will, in general, be somewhat lean, else you're ready. Shake the Worcestershire sauce and Montreal Steak Seasoning over the chicken and blend all together with your hands. Include the blue cheddar and blend once more.

Gap the meat equally and fold into three balls. Smooth into patties (I utilize a burger press) and make a slight melancholy in the focal point of every party. Flame broil to your ideal degree of doneness.

Gather: Separate the onions. Spot the cheeseburger patties on the mushrooms, top with a pat of blue cheddar margarine, and afterwards finish with 1/3 of the barbecued onions.

Notes

Nourishment Facts: Calories 708, Calories from Fat 531, % Daily Value* Fat 59g91%, Starches 10g3%, Fibre 2g8%, Protein 34g68%.

Lasagna meatballs

Yield: 8 servings

Cook time: 40 minutes

Planning time: 20 minutes

Complete-time: 60 minutes

Fixings

- For the meatballs:
- One lb. sweet or hot Italian hotdog
- 1 lb. ground throw (or turkey on the off chance that you like)

- 1/3 cup almond flour
- Two eggs
- 1 Tbsp dried parsley
- 1 tsp legitimate salt
- 1/4 tsp red pepper chips
- 1/2 tsp garlic powder
- 1/2 tsp onion powder
- 1/4 tsp dried oregano
- 1/4 cup ground Parmesan cheddar

For the dish:

- 2 cups keto marinara
- 1/2 cups entire milk mozzarella cheddar, destroyed
- 1 cup entire milk ricotta cheddar

Directions

For the meatballs:

Consolidate the entirety of the meatball fixings in a medium bowl and blend thoroughly. Structure into around thirty-two 1.5″ meatballs. Spot the meatballs on a material lined preparing sheet and heat at 375 degrees (F) for 15 minutes.

For the dish:

Spot the meatballs in a meal dish (13×9 ought to do) in a solitary layer. Pour half of the keto marinara sauce over the meatballs. Drop the ricotta cheddar by liberal teaspoonfuls uniformly over the meal. Pour the other 50% of the marinara sauce over the top. Sprinkle the mozzarella cheddar over the whole thing. Prepare for around 30 minutes at 375 degrees. Expel from the broiler and let it cool for about five minutes before serving.

NOTES

Approx. Sustenance data per serving: 494 calories, 39g fat, 4g net carbs, 31g protein.

Heavenly Beef Broccoli Recipe

Fixings

Servings: 8

Planning time: 10 minutes

Cook time: 20 minutes

The aggregate of 30 minutes

- 2 lb. of ground hamburger
- 1.5 pound. of solidified broccoli

- (2) 16 oz containers of Alfredo Sauce
- 2 T of Italian Seasoning
- 1 T of garlic powder

Headings

Ground the meat in a significant skillet with the flavouring, channel the fat. Include the broccoli and Alfredo sauce in the skillet. Cook until the broccoli is cooked. Present with a serving of mixed greens.

Wholesome actualities

40g fat, 3g net carbs, 32g protein.

Stuffed Spaghetti Squash

Fixings

- 3 lb. spaghetti squash
- 1 lb. ground hamburger
- One green pepper, diced
- One onion, diced
- Three garlic cloves, minced
- One portobello mushroom, divided and cut
- 1 (28 oz) can diced tomatoes, depleted
- Salt and pepper
- 1/2 tsp. dried thyme
- 1 tsp. dried oregano
- 1/4 tsp. cayenne
- Parmesan cheddar for garnish whenever wanted

Guidelines

Preheat grill to 400F. Wound a blade into the spaghetti squash haphazardly about multiple times to enable steam to discharge. Spot on a preparing sheet and cooking for 30-40 minutes, or until a blade can penetrate through the skin effectively. Cut into equal parts and permit to cool. Evacuate seeds. Utilizing a fork, run it inside the squash to make the spaghetti "noodles."

Filling

Warmth a large skillet over medium-high heat. Include the meat, onions, garlic, and mushrooms. Cook until chicken is caramelized. Blend in tomatoes, green pepper, salt, and pepper. Sprinkle with thyme, oregano, and cayenne. Diminish warmth and stew for 10 minutes.

Diminish stove to 350F. Include the sauce top of your readied squash parts. Sprinkle with Parmesan cheddar whenever wanted. Prepare for 10 minutes, or until warmed through and cheddar is softened.

Low Carb Slow Cooker Kickin' Chili

Planning Time: 30 minutes

Cook Time: 8 hours

Total Time: 8 hours 30 minutes

Fixings

- 2 1/2 pounds ground hamburger
- One medium red onion slashed and separated
- Five cloves garlic, minced
- Three enormous ribs of celery, diced
- 1/4 cup salted jalapeno cuts
- 6 ounces would tomato be able to glue
- 14.5 ounce can tomato and green chillies
- 14.5 ounce can stew tomatoes
- Two tablespoons Worcestershire sauce or Coconut Amines (I utilize this brand)
- Four tablespoons stew powder (I use this brand)
- Two tablespoons cumin, mounded
- Two teaspoons ocean salt
- One teaspoon garlic powder
- One teaspoon onion powder
- One teaspoon oregano
- One teaspoon dark pepper
- 1/2 teaspoon cayenne
- One inlet leaf

Directions

Cook with a low heat level.

In a large skillet over medium-high warmth, include ground meat, half of the onions, 2 Tbs. Minced garlic, and salt and pepper. When the chicken is sautéed, channel overabundance oil from skillet.

Move ground meat blend to slow cooker. Include remaining onions, garlic, celery, jalapenos, tomato glue, tomatoes and chillies (with fluid), stewed tomatoes (with liquid), Worcestershire sauce, bean stew powder, cumin, salt, cayenne, garlic powder, onion powder, oregano, dark pepper, and narrows leaf.

Mix until all fixings are very much joined. Cook on low 6-8 hours.

NOTES

Per Serving: 1 Cup

Calories: 137, Fat: 5g, Protein: 16g, Net Carbs: 4.7g.

Keto Balsamic Coated Meatloaf

Planning Time: 10 minutes

Cook Time: 50 minutes

All out Time: 60 minutes

Fixings

- For the meatloaf (or meatballs):
- 3 lbs. ground hamburger (80/20)
- 1 cup white mushrooms, minced
- Two cloves garlic, minced
- 1/2 cup onion, finely slashed
- 1/4 cup red ringer pepper, finely cleaved
- 2 Tbsp crisp parsley, finely cleaved
- 1/3 cup ground Parmesan cheddar
- 1/2 cup almond flour
- Three eggs
- 1 tsp fit salt
- 1/4 tsp ground dark pepper
- 1 tsp balsamic vinegar
- For the coating:
- 2 cups balsamic vinegar (no sugar included)
- 2 Tbsp low sugar or sugar-free ketchup
- 1 Tbsp granulated sugar substitute (Swerve, Splenda and Ideal.)

Guidelines

Join the entirety of the meatloaf fixings in a medium bowl and blend all together.

In the case of making meatballs:

Structure the meat blend into 48 mixed drink measured meatballs (around 1 inch).

Spot the meatballs on material paper or a lubed treat sheet and heat for 8-10 minutes at 375 degrees (F) or until cooked.

Add the meatballs to the coating and hurl delicately to cover. Serve hot.

In the case of making meatloaf:

Press the meat blend into two 8-9″ portion skillet and heat at 375 degrees for 30 minutes.

Expel from the broiler and pour off the more significant part of the fluid from the two dishes.

Pour 1/4 cup of coating over every one of the meatloaves and come back to the barbecue.

Heat for an additional 20 minutes.

Cool for at any rate 10 minutes before cutting and presenting with the rest of the coating.

For the coating:

Join the balsamic vinegar, ketchup, and sugar-free sugar in a little container.

Heat to the point of boiling, at that point, lessen warmth to medium-low and stew for around 20 minutes or until decreased by at any rate half and somewhat thickened and sparkly.

The coating is prepared when it's sufficiently thick to cover the rear of a spoon.

Refrigerate any additional coating for some time later.

NOTES

Inexact sustenance data:

Per 4 meatballs w/coat: 264 calories, 17g fat, 6g net carbs, 24g protein

extra 1 Tbsp coat for serving: 21 calories, 0g fat, 4g net carbs, 0g protein.

Keto Cheeseburger Casserole with Bacon

Planning Time: 20 minutes

Cook Time: 35 minutes

All out Time: 55 minutes

Servings: 12 individuals

Calories: 587 kcal

Fixings

- 2 pounds ground hamburger
- Two cloves enormous garlic
- 1/2 teaspoon onion powder
- 1 pound no sugar bacon cooked and slashed
- Eight eggs see note
- One would tomato be able to glue 6 ounces
- 1 cup substantial cream
- 1/2 teaspoon salt
- 1/4 teaspoon ground pepper
- 12 ounces ground cheddar partitioned

Guidelines

Ground hamburger with garlic and onion powder.

Channel abundance oil, at that point, spread hamburger on the base of 9×13-inch dish skillet.

Mix bacon pieces into cooked hamburger.

In a medium container, whisk together eggs, tomato glue, substantial cream, salt, and pepper until very much consolidated.

Mix 8 ounces ground cheddar into egg blend.

Pour egg blend over hamburger and bacon.

Top with staying 4 ounces of ground cheddar.

Heat at 350°F for 30-35 minutes or until brilliant darker on top.

Notes

On the off chance that you need a less eggy goulash, decrease eggs, and include more hamburger. Mushrooms, onions, and pickles are incredible include ins!

Sustenance

Serving: 1Piece

Calories: 587kcal, Carbohydrates: 4g, Protein: 29g, Fat: 49g, Saturated Fat: 22g, Cholesterol: 24mg, Sodium: 735mg, Potassium: 505mg, Sugar: 2g, Vitamin A: 965IU, Vitamin C: 3.4mg, Calcium: 255mg, Iron: 2.8mg

Extra Info

Net Carbs: 4 g | % Carbs: 2.8 % | % Protein: 20.2 % | % Fat: 77 %

Simple Taco Pie

Planning Time: 15 minutes

Cook Time: 30 minutes

All out Time: 45 minutes
Servings: 8
Calories: 370 kcal
Fixings

- 1 lb. ground meat
- 3 tbsp taco flavouring or one bundle taco flavouring
- Six huge eggs
- 1 cup overwhelming cream
- Two cloves garlic minced
- 1/2 tsp salt
- 1/4 tsp pepper
- 1 cup destroyed cheddar

Directions

Preheat stove to 350F and oil a glass or earthenware 9-inch pie container.

Dark-coloured ground meat in a large skillet over medium warmth until never again pink, around 7 minutes, separating bunches with the rear of a wooden spoon.

Include taco flavouring and mix until consolidated; at that point, diminish warmth to medium-low and cook a couple of moments longer until sauce is thickened.

Spread hamburger in arranged pie container.

In an enormous bowl, consolidate eggs, cream, garlic, salt, and pepper. Pour over meat.

Sprinkle with destroyed cheddar and heat 30 minutes, or until focus is set and cheddar is sautéed.

Evacuate and let sit 5 minutes before cutting and serving.

Top with harsh cream, cleaved tomatoes, and hacked avocado, whenever wanted.

Formula Notes

Serves 8

Each serving has 2 g of carbs.

Sustenance Facts

Sum Per Serving (1 cut (1/eighth of pie))

Calories: 370, Calories from Fat 250.

% Daily Value* Fat 27.8g43%, Sugars 2.14g1%, Fibre 0.19g1%, Protein 24.1g48%

Keto "Parmigiana" (Italian recipe)

Yield: 15 two-inch meatballs for

Serves: 3

Fixings

- For the meatballs
- 1.5lbs ground hamburger (80/20)
- 2 Tbl crisp parsley, cleaved
- 3/4 cup ground parmesan cheddar
- 1/2 cup almond flour
- Two eggs
- 1 tsp fit salt
- 1/4 tsp ground dark pepper
- 1/4 tsp garlic powder
- 1 tsp dried onion drops
- 1/4 tsp dried oregano
- 1/2 cup warm water
- For the Parmigiana
- 1 cup simple keto marinara sauce (or any sugar-free locally acquired marinara)
- 4 oz mozzarella cheddar

Guidelines

Join the entirety of the meatball fixings in a large bowl and blend well.

Structure into fifteen 2" meatballs.

Prepare at 350 degrees for 20 minutes OR fry in a large skillet over medium warmth until cooked. Professional tip – have a go at browning in bacon oil if you have any – it includes another degree of flavour. Searing produces the brilliant darker shading that appeared in the photographs above.

For the Parmigiana:

Spot the cooked meatballs in a broiler-safe dish.

Spoon around 1 Table sauce over every meatball.

Spread with around 1/4 oz of mozzarella cheddar each.

Prepare at 350 degrees (F) or 20 minutes (40 minutes if meatballs are solidified) or until warmed through, and the cheddar is brilliant.

I am topping with fresh parsley whenever wanted.

NOTES

Approx. Sustenance information per "stripped" meatball: 121 cal. 8g fat, .7g net carbs, 11g protein

Approx. Sustenance information per meatball parmigiana: 151 cal. 9g fat, 1.7g net carbs, 12g protein

Bacon Double Cheeseburger

Planning time: 10 minutes

Cook time: 20 minutes

All out Time: 30 minutes

Servings: 15 medium-large mushrooms

Fixings

- 1/2-pound lean ground hamburger
- 1/2 onion finely cleaved
- 1/4 teaspoon garlic powder
- Four tablespoons cream cheddar
- Two teaspoons ketchup
- 1/2 teaspoon yellow mustard
- Three cuts of bacon I cheat and use "prepared cooked."
- Two runs of Worcestershire sauce
- 15 mediums to enormous mushrooms
- 1/4 cup every cheddar and mozzarella cheddar or 1/2 cup cheddar

Directions

Preheat stove to 375°F.

Cook bacon until fresh, a channel on paper towels, disintegrate and put in a safe spot.

In a dish, dark-coloured ground meat, onion, and garlic powder until hamburger are cooked through. Channel any residual juices.

In the interim, haul the centre out of the mushrooms and dispose of. I utilize my strawberry/tomato huller to scratch out somewhat a higher amount of the mushrooms.

Mix cream cheddar into the meat until softened. Include ketchup, mustard, 1/4 cup cheddar, Worcestershire sauce, disintegrated bacon, and mix until joined.

On a foil-lined dish, fill each mushroom with the hamburger blend. Try not to be reluctant to heap it up high it's yummy!

Top with extra cheddar and prepare 20 minutes or until cheddar is dissolved and mushrooms are cooked.

Nourishment information:

Calories: 78

Fat: 6g, Saturated Fat: 2g

Cholesterol: 19mg, Sodium: 73mg, Potassium: 127mg, Carbohydrates: 1g, Protein: 4g, Vitamin A: 75%, Vitamin C: 0.7%, Calcium: 20%, Iron: 0.5%

Kofta Ground Beef Bowl with Garlic Tzatziki

Planning Time: 5 minutes

Cook time: 25 minutes

Absolute time: 30 MIN

Servings: 4

Fixings

- 2 Persian cucumbers
- 1/2 tsp fit salt
- One garlic clove
- 1 Pinch of salt
- 1 cup nonfat plain Greek yoghurt
- 2 tsp. olive oil
- 1/2 tsp oregano
- 1/2 lemon, juiced
- 1/4 tsp. dark pepper
- 1/4 cup red onion, diced
- 1.33 lbs. 95% lean ground hamburger
- Two garlic cloves, minced
- 1 tbsp. cumin
- 1/2 tsp red pepper drops
- 1/4 tsp cinnamon
- 1/4 tsp allspice
- 1/4 tsp coriander
- 1/4 cup parsley, minced
- Salt and pepper

Guidelines

1. To make the tzatziki: Use a crate grater to grind the cucumber. Sprinkle salt and let it be for 20 minutes. The salt will evacuate a portion of the dampness. Utilizing a paper towel or cheesecloth, crush out as much moisture as you can from the cucumber. In the interim, using the rear of your blade and spot of salt, smash garlic into the glue. When the cucumbers are prepared, blend in the yoghurt, olive oil, lemon juice, squashed garlic, oregano, pepper, and salt. Mix and refrigerate.

2. For the meat: Warmth the olive oil over medium-high warmth. Include the onion and cook for 2-3 minutes. Include the hamburger and cook, separating it with a wooden spoon, for 3-4 minutes. Include the garlic and the entirety of the spiced and keep on cooking for 4-5 minutes until meat is cooked through. Balance in the parsley and season with salt and pepper—Cook for 1-2 additional minutes.

3. To gather the dishes: Choose your preferred grain or cauliflower rice. Top with ground hamburger and garlic tzatziki. At that point, include your preferred cooked or new vegetables. I like to serve mine with an Israeli plate of mixed greens.

Calories 297 from Fat 45

% Daily Value *

Complete Fat 12g19%

Soaked Fat 4g20%

Monounsaturated Fat 3g

Polyunsaturated Fat 1g

Cholesterol 94mg31%

Sodium 569mg25%

Complete Carbohydrate 8g2%

Dietary Fiber 2g7%

Sugars 3g

Protein 39.

Keto Salisbury Steak with Mushroom Gravy

Planning Time: 10 minutes

Cook time: 20

All out time: 30 minutes

Servings: 6

Fixings

- For the Salisbury Steaks:
- 2 lbs. ground toss (80/20)
- 3/4 cup almond flour
- 1 Tbsp crisp parsley slashed
- 1/4 cup hamburger juices
- 1 Tbsp Worcestershire sauce
- 1/2 tsp garlic powder
- 1 Tbsp dried onion drops
- 1/2 tsp fit salt

- 1/2 tsp ground dark pepper
- For the sauce:
- 2 Tbsp margarine
- 2 Tbsp bacon oil (or margarine)
- 2 cups cut catch mushrooms
- 1 cup chopped yellow onions
- 1/2 tsp Worcestershire sauce
- 1/2 cup hamburger juices
- 1/4 cup harsh cream
- salt and pepper to taste

Guidelines

For the Salisbury Steaks:

Join the entirety of the steak fixings in a medium measuring bowl and blend well.

Structure into six oval patties, around 1 inch thick, and spot them on a treat sheet.

Prepare in a preheated 375-degree (F) stove for 18 minutes.

For the sauce:

Dissolve the spread and bacon fat (if utilizing) in a large skillet.

Include the mushrooms and cook medium-high warmth until brilliant dark coloured (around 3 minutes for each side.)

Include the onions and cook for 5 minutes over medium heat until bright and delicate.

Include the juices and the Worcestershire sauce, mix and cook for 3 minutes, blending to scratch any bits off of the base of the dish.

Include the harsh cream, mix well, and expel from the warmth. (if you need a thicker sauce, you can cook it on low for five additional minutes to consolidate it.)

Season with salt and pepper to taste.

Serve over the warm Salisbury Steaks with additional parsley for decorating whenever wanted.

NOTES

If anyone needs sustenance information independently:

1 Salisbury Steak: 354 calories, 24g fat, 2.5g net carbs, 30g protein

1/3 cup sauce: 103 calories, 10g fat, 2.5g net carbs, 2g protein

GROUND BEEF AND SAUERKRAUT LOW-CARB SOUP

Servings: 8
Planning time: 15 minutes
Cook time: 1 hour 15 minutes
absolute time: 1 hour 30 minutes
Fixings

* 1 lb. ground meat (see notes)
* 2 tsp. olive oil
* 2 cups custom made chicken stock (see notes)
* 2 14 oz. jars meat stock (see notes)
* 1 14.5 oz. can dice tomatoes
* 1 14 oz. can sauerkraut with (see notes)
* 1 T sugar of your decision
* 1 T Worcestershire sauce (see notes)
* Four dried narrows leave
* 3 T minced parsley (see notes)
* 1 tsp. dried scoured sage
* One medium onion slashed little
* 1 T minced garlic (or less in case you're not unreasonably enamoured with garlic)
* 1-2 cups water (if necessary)
* salt and pepper to taste

Directions

In an overwhelming skillet, heat 1 tsp. Olive oil, include ground hamburger and dark-coloured well, breaking into little smithereens with turner. This will take ten minutes; however, don't surge the sautéing step.

While ground meat tans, join chicken stock, hamburger stock, canned tomatoes with juice, sauerkraut with milk, sugar of your decision, Worcestershire sauce, cove leaves, parsley, and sage in a huge stockpot. Bring to a low stew.

At the point when meat is very much cooked, add to soup in the pot. Deglaze dish with a touch of the soup fluid, scratching off any caramelized bits, and add to soup.

Crash skillet and include other 1-2 tsp — olive oil. Saute onions 2-3 minutes, until beginning to mellow, at that point add garlic and saute 1-2 minutes more.

Add to soup, decrease heat under soup pot and let soup stew at low warmth around 60 minutes.

Following 60 minutes, taste for flavouring and include water if soup appears to be excessively substantial. Stew 15 minutes more if including water.

Season to taste with fresh ground dark pepper (and somewhat salt whenever wanted) before serving. Serve hot, with sharp cream whenever desired.

NOTES

I would utilize ground meat with under 10% fat. If you don't have custom made chicken stock utilize one can (14 oz. can) chicken soup and a little water. Start with two jars hamburger soup and include somewhat more whenever wanted. Use packaged sauerkraut on the off chance that you like. Use Gluten-Free Worcestershire Sauce (subsidiary connection) if necessary. You can utilize 1-2 T dried parsley on the off chance that you would prefer not to purchase new parsley.

Nutritional facts

Calories: 222

Total fat: 12g

Saturated fat: 4g

Unsaturated fat: 6g

Cholesterol: 52mg

Sodium: 995mg

Carbohydrates: 9g

Fiber: 3g

Sugar: 4g

Protein: 19g

Cauliflower and Ground Beef Hash

Planning time: 5 minutes

Cook time: 20 minutes

All out time: 25 minutes

Fixings

- 16 oz. sack solidified cauliflower defrosted and depleted
- 1 lb. lean ground meat
- 2 c. cheddar
- 1 tsp. garlic powder
- salt and pepper to taste

Directions

Dark-coloured the ground meat over medium warmth and channel the oil.

Add it back to the container alongside the cauliflower, garlic, salt, and pepper. Cook and mix until cauliflower are delicate.

Include cheddar top of the cauliflower and meat blend. Go warmth to low, spread dish with a head, and enable cheddar to dissolve.

Sustenance Facts

Serves 6

Sum Per Serving

Calories   263

% Daily Value*

All out Fat 15g   23%

Cholesterol 82.5mg 27%

Sodium 701.7mg   29%

All out Carbohydrate 5.1g   2%

Dietary Fiber 1.8g   7%

Sugars 1.9g

Protein 26.8g   54%

Nutrient A 9%Vitamin C 61%

MEATLOAF CUPCAKES

Planning time: 10 minutes

Cook time: 30 minutes

All out time: 40 minutes

Fixings

- One onion diced finely
- 700 g ground/mince hamburger
- Two eggs - medium gently beat
- salt and pepper to taste
- 100 g destroyed/ground cheddar
- Instances of Flavorings
- Two cuts bacon diced
- bunch crisp basil
- bunch crisp parsley
- 4 tbsp sundried tomatoes diced
- 2 tsp dried oregano

Guidelines

Base Recipe

Blend the diced onion, meat, eggs and salt, and pepper.

Include your selection of seasonings and flavourings. I have given one model, however, to investigate a colossal scope of thoughts.

Combine every one of the fixings with your hands and spot a little bunch of the meatloaf blend into the biscuit plate. Press tenderly, not very hard, else they will transform into meatballs.

Spread with the ground cheddar and sprinkle with ground parmesan whenever wanted.

Cook at 180C/350F

Notes

Mince/ground meat can be hamburger, pork, turkey, or chicken of your decision.

Sustenance will differ as indicated by which meat you pick and how lean it is.

Attempt to pick the medium-fat meat. Generally, an excessive amount of fat will render out.

Sum Per Serving

Calories 221 Calories from Fat 155

% Daily Value*

Fat 17.2g26%

Sugars 1g0%

Fiber 0.4g2%

Sugar 0.7g1%

Protein 15.2g30%

* Percent Daily Values depend on a 2000 calorie diet.

Cumin Spiced Beef Wraps

Planning time: 15 minutes

Cook time: 10 minutes

Absolute time: 25 minutes

Yield: makes 2 Servings

Fixings

- 1–2 tbsp coconut oil
- 1/4 onion, diced little
- 2/3 lb. ground meat
- One red chime pepper, diced little
- 2 tbsp cilantro, cleaved
- 1 tsp ginger, minced
- Four cloves garlic, minced

- 2 tsp cumin
- Salt and pepper, to taste
- Eight huge cabbage leaves (savoy cabbage or Napa cabbage)

Directions

Spot 1-2 tbsp of coconut oil into a skillet and sauté the onions, ground hamburger, and peppers on medium warmth.

At the point when the ground meat is cooked, include the cilantro, ginger, garlic, cumin, salt, and pepper to taste.

Fill an enormous pot 3/4 full with water and heat to the point of boiling.

Utilizing tongs, whiten each cabbage leaf in the bubbling water (put each sheet into the bubbling water for 20 seconds). At that point, dive each leaf into some virus water before depleting and setting onto a plate.

Spoon the meat blend onto every lettuce leaf and crease into a tube.

NOTES

Per Serving – Calories: 375

Fat: 26g

Protein: 30g

Total Carbs: 6g

Fiber: 2g

Net Carbs: 4g

Low-Carb Grain-Free Meatloaf

Yield: 10 servings

Planning time: 25 Minutes

Cook time: 1 hour 30 minutes

Complete-time: 1 Hour 55 minutes

Fixings

- 2 lbs. ground meat (see notes)
- 1 19.5 oz. Pkg. hot turkey Italian Sausage
- 1 14.5 oz. would petite be able to dice tomatoes, depleted and cleaved
- 2 T dried hacked onion
- 1 T garlic powder
- 1 T dried basil
- 1 T dried parsley
- 1/2 cup flaxseed dinner (see notes)

- 1 tsp. Vege-Sal (see notes)
- 1 T ground fennel
- Two eggs somewhat are beaten

Directions

Preheat stove to 375 F.

Splash simmering racks or portion dish with non-stick shower.

Expel ground meat and turkey frankfurter joins from the fridge and let come to room temperature.

Channel canned tomatoes into a colander put in the sink. At the point when they are well-depleted, put them on cutting board and leave them somewhat littler.

In a bowl, consolidate dried onion, garlic powder, dried basil, dried parsley, flaxseed meal, Vege-Sal or salt, and ground fennel. (I intentionally utilized dried herbs since I wasn't adding many folios to the meatloaf, and I didn't need included dampness.)

Crush turkey frankfurter out of housings in little pieces and add to the blending bowl.

Kick things off hamburger into pieces and spot in the same bowl.

Include cleaved tomatoes, and eggs to meat blend and utilize your hands to consolidate well.

Attempt to blend the meat enough to get flavours and eggs equitably appropriated without over-blending shape meat into two portions.

Prepare until the meatloaf is very much done and shows 165F on an Instant Read Meat Thermometer (offshoot connect) or if you don't have a meat thermometer cut one open and ensure within is done.

Sustenance INFORMATION

Sum per serving:

Calories: 409

Total fat: 25g

Saturated fat: 8g

Unsaturated fat: 13g

Cholesterol: 171mg

Sodium: 487mg

Carbohydrates: 3g

Fiber: 2g

Sugar: 0g
Protein: 41g
Low Carb Pepperoni Pizza Meatballs
Yield: 5 servings of 3 meatballs each
All-out time: 60 minutes
Fixings
- For the meatballs:
- 1 lb. ground hamburger (80/20)
- One egg
- 1/3 cup almond flour
- 1/2 cup destroyed crude zucchini
- 1/4 cup pepperoni, slashed
- 1/3 cup parmesan cheddar, ground
- 1/2 tsp garlic powder
- 1/2 tsp onion powder
- 1/4 tsp fit salt
- 1/8 tsp ground dark pepper
- 2 Tbsp olive oil for singing
- To serve:
- 1 cup ten Free)">Easy Keto Marinara Sauce
- 1/2 cup destroyed entire milk mozzarella
- 15 cuts pepperoni

Guidelines
To make the meatballs:
Join the entirety of meatball fixings (aside from the olive oil) in a medium bowl and blend. Structure into 15 meatballs. Warmth the oil in a nonstick dish and fry the meatballs until brilliant dark coloured – around 3 minutes for each side. Expel and spot on a paper towel-lined plate.
To serve:
Spot the meatballs in a broiler verification dish. Spoon the sauce equitably over every meatball—top with destroyed mozzarella cheddar, and a cut of pepperoni. Heat for 10 minutes at 375 degrees, or set under the oven for 2 – 3 minutes until the cheddar is dissolved and the pepperoni is getting fresh. Serve hot.
NOTES
Approx. Sustenance information per serving: 380 calories, 28g fat, 3g net carbs, 27g protein.

Low Carb Big Mac Casserole
Planning time: 15 minutes
Cook time: 20 minutes
All out time: 35 minutes
Yield: Makes six servings
Fixings
•	2 pounds ground hamburger
•	Two tablespoons minced onion pieces
•	One tablespoon Worcestershire sauce
•	Two cloves garlic, minced
•	ocean salt and dark pepper, to taste
•	2 cups destroyed sharp cheddar, partitioned
•	1 cup destroyed mozzarella cheddar
•	1 cup Russian Dressing, partitioned (get the formula here)
•	1 cup dill pickle cuts, around 20
•	Two tablespoons toasted sesame seeds
•	One enormous head of romaine lettuce, cleaved
Guidelines
Preheat grill to 350°
In a large skillet over medium warmth, dark-coloured the ground hamburger, minced onion drops, garlic, Worcestershire sauce, ocean salt, and dark pepper. Channel overabundance oil and move to a large goulash dish.
To the ground meat, include 1 cup sharp cheddar, mozzarella cheddar, and 3/4 cup Russian dressing. Blend until all fixings are very much consolidated. Level down into a decent and even minimal layer. Top with pickle cuts.
Sprinkle the rest of the cup of sharp cheddar over the top. Sprinkle the sesame seeds over the cheddar.
Heat for 20 minutes. Turn the stove up to a high cook and prepare for an additional 5 minutes.
Plate each serving over a bed of destroyed lettuce and top with staying Russian dressing.
NOTES
5.8g net carbs per serving
Nourishment
Calories: 556
Fat: 51g

Carbohydrates: 8.8g
Fibre: 3g
Protein: 45g

Ground Beef Jerky

Planning Time: 30 minutes
Cook time: 8 hours
Complete-time: 8 hours 30 minutes
Servings: 32 strips
Calories: 186kcal

Fixings

- 3 pounds ground meat or venison
- Five teaspoons garlic powder
- Four teaspoons ocean salt
- Four teaspoons new ground pepper
- One tablespoon fluid smoke

Directions

Consolidate all fixings in a large blending bowl.

Utilizing a jerky weapon, press light strips onto dehydrator racks. Or then again, roll flimsy between material paper, cut into strips and spot on shelves.

Dry out for 7-12 hours until dry and fresh.

Store as long as seven days in cooler or freeze for longer stockpiling.

Notes

Makes 16 servings (2 strips each)

Sustenance per serving (2 pieces): 0.5g net carb

Nourishment
Serving: 2g
Calories: 186kcal
Carbohydrates: 0.6g
Protein: 16g
Fat: 12.8g
Sodium: 640mg
Fiber: 0.1g

Meat Veggie Chili

Planning time: 10 minutes
Cook time: 30 minutes
Absolute time: 40 minutes
Yield: 8 servings

Fixings

- 1/2 pounds ground meat
- Two cloves garlic, cleaved
- Two tablespoons (30 ml) oil
- 1/2 cups onion, diced, around one huge onion
- 1/2 cup cleaved celery, around one stalk
- 1/2 cups carrots, peeled and diced, around four medium carrots
- Two tablespoons bean stew powder
- One teaspoon ground cumin
- One teaspoon oregano
- One teaspoon salt
- 1/4 teaspoon cayenne pepper (discretionary)
- 4 cups zucchinis, diced, around 2–3 medium zucchinis
- 1 15-ounce would tomato be able to puree or tomato sauce
- One 15-ounce can dice tomatoes

Directions

In your prepared skillet or 5-6-quart large cast iron pot, dark-coloured meat and garlic. Cook over medium warmth until beef is thoroughly cooked and sautéed. Channel off overabundance fat put in a safe spot.

Include oil, onions, celery, carrots, and seasonings to the skillet and cook until translucent over medium-high warmth, around 5-7 minutes. When onions are brilliant, and veggies are halfway cooked, include zucchini and cook for 2 minutes, ensuring you mix everything admirably.

Include cooked meat, tomato puree/sauce, and tomatoes into the pot and mix well. Heat everything to the point of boiling, blending as often as possible, decrease warmth, and stew for 20 minutes.

Mind the stunning blend occasionally and mix. Serve right away.

Sustenance

Serving Size: 1 serving

Calories: 294Fat: 10.3g

Carbohydrates: 27.3g

Protein: 26g

Low-Carb Spaghetti with Zoodles

Planning Time: 15 minutes
Cook Time
20 minutes
All out Time
35 minutes
servings: 3
Fixings
- One onion finely slashed
- Two cloves garlic squashed
- 500 g mince/ground hamburger
- 400 g tinned/canned cut tomatoes
- determination of crisp or dried Italian herbs - I utilize the accompanying
- 1 tbsp dried rosemary
- 1 tbsp dried oregano
- 1 tbsp dried sage
- 1 tbsp dried basil
- 1 tbsp dried marjoram
- salt and pepper to taste

Directions

In a huge pot. Tenderly fry the onion and garlic in oil until relaxed however not overcooked.

Include the mince/ground meat and keep on broiling blending persistently to separate the mince/ground hamburger. Fry until all the chicken is cooked and sautéed.

Include some herbs, flavours, and tomato.

Mix at and stew for 15 minutes while you cook the zoodles.

Serve in a bowl with zoodles and cheddar or parmesan sprinkled on top.

Nourishment Facts
Low Carb Spaghetti Bolognese
Sum Per Serving   (1 serving)
Calories 318 Calories from Fat 153
% Daily Value*
Fat 17g26%
Starches 13g4%
Fiber 4g17%
Sugar 7g8%
Protein 30g

Keto Bacon Cheeseburger
Yield: 12 meatballs (4 servings)
Complete-time: 1hour.
Fixings
- For the Meatballs:
- 1 lb ground meat (I like 80/20 for these)
- One egg
- 1/4 cup almond flour
- 3/4 tsp salt
- 1/4 tsp ground dark pepper
- 1/2 tsp garlic powder
- 1/4 cup hacked crude bacon (from the greasy finishes)
- bacon fat to cook the meatballs in

For the Sauce:
- 1/4 cup mayonnaise
- 1 Tbsp sugar-free ketchup
- 1 tsp Dijon mustard
- 1 Tbsp dill pickle juice
- To Serve:
- 3 oz cheddar (or other) cheddar
- 4 cups chunk of ice lettuce, destroyed
- Three cuts of bacon, cooked and broken into 12 pieces

Guidelines

Join the entirety of the meatball fixings in a medium bowl and blend thoroughly. Structure into 12 meatballs. Fry in a non-stick dish in the held bacon fat (or utilize the oil of your decision) for around 4 minutes for the first side. Turn them over and cover each with a cut of cheddar—Cook for an extra 4 minutes, or until done just as you would prefer. Expel from the warmth, and top every meatball with a bit of bacon.

For the Sauce:

Consolidate the entirety of the sauce fixings in a little bowl and whisk together until smooth.

To Serve:

Spot 1 cup of destroyed ice burg lettuce on a plate. Top with three meatballs and shower with around 1/2 Tablespoons of sauce.

NOTES

Inexact nourishment data per serving:

One meatball: 160 calories, 11g fat, .25g net carbs, 14g protein
Three meatballs w/sauce and lettuce: 591 calories, 45g fat, 1.5g net carbs, 42g protein.

Low Carb Swedish Meatballs

Planning time: 15 minutes
Cook time: 25 minutes
Absolute time: 40 minutes
Servings: 15 individuals
Calories: 294kcal

Fixings

- Meatballs
- 2 pounds lean ground meat
- Two huge eggs
- 4 ounces onion, minced and sautéed until delicate
- 1/4 cup overwhelming cream
- One tablespoon Worcestershire sauce
- One tablespoon Montreal Steak Seasoning
- One tablespoon Low carb dark coloured sugar or your preferred sugar
- One teaspoon unadulterated ground chipotle pepper flavouring
- 1/2 teaspoon pepper
- 1/4 teaspoon salt
- 1/4 teaspoon allspice
- 1/4 teaspoon nutmeg
- Two tablespoons olive oil isolated

Sauce

- 4 ounces cream cheddar
- 1/2 cups unsalted hamburger juices
- 1 cup substantial cream
- Two tablespoons Brandy
- Two teaspoons Dijon mustard
- Two teaspoons Worcestershire sauce
- 1/4 teaspoon salt
- 1/8 teaspoon pepper
- decorate with slashed parsley

Guidelines

Meatballs: In a large skillet, heat two teaspoons of oil over medium-high warmth until hot. Include the minced onions and saute until delicate.

Put the entirety of elements for meatballs into an enormous bowl and blend in with hand blender until joined and light and feathery.

Utilizing a tablespoon measure, scoop the meatball blend, fold into a ball, and spot onto a foil-lined sheet skillet. I like to keep my hands apply oil, so the meatballs don't adhere to my hands. Two tablespoons of oil in a little bowl is a bounty. By estimating cautiously, you ought to get around 60 meatballs.

In a similar dish where the onions were sautéed, heat around two teaspoons of oil over medium-high warmth. Include half of the meatballs turning everyone three times, at around 2 minutes for each side.

Evacuate the meatballs to the sheet skillet, lift half of the foil and spot them on the perfect sheet container. Include the remainder of the oil to the saute container and cook the staying half of the meatballs. Expel the meatballs to the sheet skillet. Mood killer, the warmth under the saute container.

Cream Sauce: Heat the cream cheddar in the microwave for one moment. Pour the two tablespoons of schnapps and 1/4 cup of the meat stock into the container, turning the warmth to medium-high. Scrape up the entirety of the darker bits on the base and sides of the box. Include the cream cheddar and split it up and attempt to liquefy it decently well. Include the cream and mix. Put the sauce from the dish into a blender and include the remainder of the hamburger soup. Mix until smooth and add it back to the container. Include the Worcestershire sauce and Dijon Mustard. Stew the sauce until it decreases smooth and add it back to the dish. Include the Worcestershire sauce and Dijon Mustard. Stew the sauce until it diminishes and thickens just as you would prefer, 5 - 10 minutes. Change flavouring. It is trimming with hacked parsley.

Utilize a looser sauce for hors d'oeuvres (like in a simmering pot) and a thicker sauce for supper.

Notes

Serving size is four meatballs each for a starter.

On the off-chance filling in as a dish with the sauce (6 meatballs) Cal: 440, Fat: 38, Carbohydrates: 3, Fiber: follow, Protein: 20.

Sustenance Facts

Low Carb Swedish Meatballs

Sum per serving:

Calories 294

Calories from fat 225

% Daily Value* Fat 25g38%

Sugars 2g1%

Protein 13g26%

Low-Carb Sriracha Beef Lettuce Wraps

Yield: 4 servings

Planning time: 15 minutes

Cook time: 10 minutes

Complete-time: 25 minutes

Fixings

• 2 tsp. cooking oil of your decision

• 1 lb. ground meat

• 1 T fish sauce (see notes)

• 1-2 T Sriracha Sauce (contingent upon how much warmth you need)

• 2 T water

• get-up-and-go from one huge lime

• juice from one huge lime (see notes)

• 1/4 cup daintily cut green onion

• 1/2 cup packed cilantro (see notes)

• Two little heads chunk of ice lettuce washed and cut into cups

Directions

Warmth the oil in an overwhelming skillet over medium-high heat, at that point cook the hamburger until it's cooked through and beginning to dark-coloured, breaking separated with a turner as it boils.

While meat cooks, combine the fish sauce, Sriracha Sauce (subsidiary connection), and water in a little bowl.

Get-up-and-go the skin of the lime and crush the juice. (You may require two limes to get enough squeeze but also utilize the get-up-and-go from one lime.)

Meagerly cut the green onions and cleave the cilantro.

Most icy mass lettuce needn't bother with washing, yet expel the outer leaves. Cut out the centre and slice the lettuce into quarters to make "cups" to hold the meat blend.

At the point when the hamburger is done, include the Sriracha Sauce blend and let it sizzle until the water has dissipated, mixing a couple of times to get the flavour blended through the meat.

Mood killer the warmth and mix in the lime pizzazz, lime juice, cut green onions, and slashed cilantro.

Serve meat blend with icy mass lettuce leaves to load up with meat and fold over it, to be eaten with your hands.

NOTES

I utilize Red Boat Fish Sauce (subsidiary connection) for this formula, which is sans gluten and Keto. You need around 1/2 T lime juice, so use two limes if necessary. In case you're not a cilantro fan, use all the more meagerly cut green onion. This was unquestionably still acceptable when the meat blend was kept in the ice chest and warmed for an exceptionally brief time in the microwave, yet I enjoyed it best newly made.

Sustenance information: yield: 4 serving size: 1

Sum per serving:

Calories: 396

Total fat: 22g

Saturated fat: 8g

Unsaturated fat: 11g

 Cholesterol: 101mg

Sodium: 711mg

Carbohydrates: 8g

Fiber: 2g

Sugar: 11g

Protein: 32g

Jamaican Meat Pies

Yield: 12 little hand pies

all-out time 60 minutes

Fixings

- For the filling:
- 1/2 lb. ground pork
- 1/2 lb. ground hamburger (85% lean)

- One small onion, cleaved
- Three cloves of garlic, cleaved
- 1/2 cup water
- One scotch cap or two habaneros
- 1 tsp Jamaican curry powder
- 1 tsp dried thyme
- 2 tsp ground coriander
- 2 tsp ground cumin
- 1/2 tsp allspice
- 1/2 tsp turmeric
- 1/8 tsp ground cloves
- 1 tsp garlic powder
- 1/4 tsp stevia powder
- salt and pepper to taste
- 2 Tbsp margarine
- For the outside layer:
- 6 oz cream cheddar, mellowed
- 4 Tbsp margarine, mollified
- 1 tsp turmeric
- 1/4 tsp salt
- 1/4 tsp stevia
- 1/2 tsp heating powder
- 1/2 cup coconut flour
- 1/2 cup processed flax supper
- 2 Tbsp cold water

Guidelines

To make the filling, add the meat to a saute skillet over medium warmth.

Puree the onion, garlic, scotch cap or habaneros, and water in a blender or enchantment shot. Empty the blend into the meat while still crude and mix it in to help prevent the meat from bunching. Add the entirety of your flavours to the meat while cooking. When thoroughly cooked and the more significant part of the water has dissipated, taste and alter flavouring to your inclination.

Include the spread and mix until liquefied and mixed into your meat blend. Expel from the warmth.

To make the batter: Blend the margarine and cream cheddar until soft.

In a different bowl, consolidate the flax, coconut flour, preparing powder, salt, stevia, and turmeric until mixed.

Add the dry fixings to the cream cheddar and spread blend, trailed by the water – mix until a solid batter structure.

Partition the batter into 12 balls somewhere in the range of one and two crawls in the distance across. Spot a ball onto a bit of material paper and spread it with another bit of material. Fold into a meagre hover around 4-5 creeps in width. Spot a couple of tablespoons of the meat blend on one portion of the circle and afterwards overlay over the other half and press or pleat to seal. (You may need to utilize a spatula to discharge the battery from the material to overlap it over.)

Spot the pie on preparing sheet shrouded in plastic and rehash with the remainder of the batter balls.

Heat in a 350-degree (F) stove for 25 minutes or until fresh.

Sustenance

Serving Size: 1 meat pie

Calories: 296

Fat: 24gCarbohydrates: 3g net Protein: 12g

Spinach Tomato Meatza Pizza

Planning Time: 8 minutes

Cook time: 22 minutes

All out time: 30 minutes

Servings: 8

Calories: 344kcal

Fixings

- Two eggs
- 1/2 cup parmesan cheddar ground
- Two teaspoons Italian seasonings
- One teaspoon garlic powder
- One teaspoon salt
- 2 pounds ground hamburger
- Two tomatoes
- 9 ounces solidified cleaved spinach cooked and depleted
- 2 cups mozzarella cheddar destroyed

Guidelines

Beat the eggs with the parmesan cheddar and all seasonings.

Include the ground hamburger and blend until all around consolidated.

Spread the blend onto a large preparing sheet with sides (a jam moves dish functions admirably).

The blend doesn't need to fill the base of the dish; I made adjusted finishes.

Prepare for around 20 minutes in a 450-degree F stove.

Expel from the stove and channel off any oil.

Spot cut tomatoes and spinach on top at that point sprinkle with mozzarella cheddar.

Profit to the stove for a high rack close to the oven. Sear until cheddar is softened and darker.

Nourishment
Serving: 296g
Calories: 344kcal
Carbohydrates: 4.1g
Protein: 47.3g
Fat: 14.9g
Saturated Fat: 7.1g
Cholesterol: 162mg
Sodium: 643mg
Potassium: 730mg
Fiber: 1.2g
Sugar: 1.1g
Vitamin A: 3350IU
Vitamin C: 18.2mg
Calcium: 130mg
Iron: 22.5mg
Low Carb Swedish Meatballs
Prep time: 10 minutes
Cook time: 20 minutes
Total Time: 30 minutes
Servings: 15 people
Calories: 294kcal
Fixings
- Meatballs
- 2 pounds lean ground meat
- Two huge eggs
- 4 ounces onion, minced and sautéed until delicate

- 1/4 cup overwhelming cream
- One tablespoon Worcestershire sauce
- One tablespoon Montreal Steak Seasoning
- One tablespoon Low carb dark coloured sugar or your preferred sugar
- One teaspoon unadulterated ground chipotle pepper flavouring
- 1/2 teaspoon pepper
- 1/4 teaspoon salt
- 1/4 teaspoon allspice
- 1/4 teaspoon nutmeg
- Two tablespoons olive oil partitioned
- Sauce
- 4 ounces cream cheddar
- 1/2 cups unsalted meat soup
- 1 cup overwhelming cream
- Two tablespoons Brandy
- Two teaspoons Dijon mustard
- Two teaspoons Worcestershire sauce
- 1/4 teaspoon salt
- 1/8 teaspoon pepper
- embellish with hacked parsley

Directions

Meatballs: In a considerable skillet, heat two teaspoons of oil over medium-high warmth until hot. Include the minced onions and saute until delicate.

Put the entirety of elements for meatballs into a considerable bowl and blend with a hand blender until joined and light and fleecy.

Utilizing a tablespoon measure, scoop the meatball blend, fold into a ball, and spot onto a foil-lined sheet container. I like to keep my hands oiled, so the meatballs don't adhere to my hands. Two tablespoons of oil in a little bowl is a bounty. By estimating cautiously, you ought to get around 60 meatballs.

In a similar dish wherein, the onions were sautéed, heat around two teaspoons of oil over medium-high warmth. Include half of the meatballs turning everyone three times, at around 2 minutes for each side.

Evacuate the meatballs to the sheet skillet, lift half of the foil and spot them on the perfect sheet dish. Include the remainder of the oil to the saute skillet and cook the staying half of the meatballs. Evacuate the meatballs to the sheet skillet. Mood killer, the warmth under the saute container.

Cream Sauce: Heat the cream cheddar in the microwave for one moment. Pour the two tablespoons of schnapps and 1/4 cup of the hamburger stock into the skillet, turning the warmth to medium-high. Scrape up the entirety of the dark-coloured bits on the base and sides of the dish. Include the cream cheddar and split it up and attempt to soften it decently well. Include the cream and mix. Put the sauce from the plate into a blender and include the remainder of the hamburger stock. Mix until smooth and add it back to the skillet. Include the Worcestershire sauce and Dijon Mustard. Stew the sauce until it diminishes and thickens just as you would prefer, 5 - 10 minutes. Change flavouring. I am trimming with cleaved parsley.

Utilize a looser sauce for canapés (like in a simmering pot) and a thicker sauce for supper.

Notes

Serving size is four meatballs each for a starter.

On the off-chance filling in as a dish with the sauce (6 meatballs) Cal: 440, Fat: 38, Carbohydrates: 3, Fiber: follow, Protein: 20

*I recommend serving over steamed zucchini noodles or cauliflower rice since the supper is so calorie thick.

Nourishment Facts

Sum Per Serving

Calories: 294

Calories from fat: 225

% Daily Value*

Fat 25g38%

Starches 2g1%

Protein 13g26%

American Goulash

Planning time: 5 minutes

Cook time: 20 minutes

Complete-time: 25 minutes

Servings: 5 servings
Calories: 223kcal
Fixings

- 1/2 pounds lean ground meat
- Salt and pepper
- 3/4 cup Bell pepper diced - around 2 oz
- 1/4 cup Onion hacked - around 1 oz
- 2 cups cauliflower about 8oz, broken into florets
- 14 ounces diced tomatoes one can - channel and spare the juice
- 14 ounces Water
- One tablespoon tomato glue
- 1/4 teaspoon garlic powder discretionary
- One parcel Monk fruit single-size serving, pretty much to taste

Guidelines

Darker the ground meat in an overwhelming skillet.
Include the ringer pepper and onion.
Saute until the vegetables are delicate.
Include the cauliflower.
Include the spared tomato squeeze and water.
Bring to a stew and spread.
Stew for 5 minutes, or until the cauliflower is delicate.
Reveal and stew a couple of moments more to lessen the fluid in the dish.
Mix in the tomato glue, tomatoes, and garlic powder in case you're utilizing it.
Taste and include the monk fruit on the off chance that you'd like it to have somewhat more sweetness.
Serve.
You can likewise quantify this into single 1 cup servings and refrigerate or freeze for some other time.

Notes

Carbs: 7.4
Net carbs: 4.8
Calories: 287
Five portions of 1 cup

Cabbage Lasagna Recipe

Planning time: 10 minutes

Cook time 35 minutes
All out time 45 minutes
Servings: 20 individuals
Calories: 451kcal
Fixings

- One head cabbage
- 3 lbs. ricotta cheddar
- 1/2 cups parmesan cheddar ground
- 1/4 cup dried parsley discretionary
- Three enormous eggs
- 2 pounds ground meat caramelized
- 40 ounces marinara sauce with no sugar included
- 32 ounces crisp mozzarella cheddar cut or destroyed
- 1/4 cup parmesan ground (discretionary)

Guidelines

Cautiously expel leaves from cabbage head.

Parboil leaves in salted bubbling water for 5-10 minutes. Channel and evacuate abundant water with a towel.

Blend ricotta and parmesan cheddar with eggs and parsley (if utilizing). Put in a safe spot.

Mix marinara sauce into sautéed meat.

Spread around 3/4 cup sauce onto the base of 11×15-inch preparing containers.

Spot a layer of cooked cabbage leaves over the sauce.

Spread half ricotta cheddar blend over cabbage leaves.

Top cheddar blend with a large portion of the rest of the sauce.

Spread sauce with a large portion of the mozzarella cheddar.

Rehash layers.

Finish off with extra parmesan cheddar whenever wanted.

Prepare 350F for around 25 moment

Notes

Nourishment

Serving: 379g
Calories: 451kcal
Carbohydrates: 9g
Protein: 27g
Fat: 34g
Saturated Fat: 17g
Cholesterol: 131mg

Sodium: 511mg
Fiber: 1g
Sugar: 3g

Extra Info
Net Carbs: 8 g | % Carbs: 7.2 % | % Protein: 24.2 % | % Fat: 68.6 %

Cauliflower Rice Taco Bowls
Yield: 6 servings
Complete-time: 35-38 minutes
Planning time: 10 minutes
Cook time: 25-28 minutes
Fixings:
Meat Ingredients:
- 2 tsp. olive oil
- 1 lb. ground meat
- salt and new ground pepper to taste
- 2 tsp. Spike Seasoning (or utilize another generally useful flavouring blend)
- 1 T Kalyn's Taco Seasoning (or utilize an obtained taco flavouring)
- 1/2 cup tomato salsa, see notes
- 1/2 cup water
- 1 4 oz. can dice green Anaheim chiles with juice

Besting Ingredients:
- 1 6 oz. can dark olives, depleted and cut down the middle
- Two medium avocados, diced
- 1 T lime juice (for avocados)
- 1 cup diced cherry tomatoes
- 1 cup ground Mexican Blend cheddar
- CAULIFLOWER RICE INGREDIENTS:
- 2 12 oz. bundles solidified cauliflower rice (see notes)
- 2 tsp. olive oil
- garlic cloves for flavouring the oil, discretionary
- One enormous Poblano chile pepper (see notes)
- 1 cup cut green onions
- salt and pepper to taste

Headings:
Warmth 2 tsp. Olive oil in a medium-sized skillet, include the ground meat, season with salt and a little dark pepper, and cook over medium-high heat until the hamburger is pleasantly caramelized. Utilize the turner or a potato masher to break the meat separated as it cooks.

At the point when meat is well-sautéed, include Spike Seasoning (subsidiary connection), Kalyn's Taco Seasoning, salsa, water, and diced green chiles and stew until the majority of the fluid has dissipated.

While the meat cooks, channelled the olives and cut down the middle, cut up avocados and hurl with the lime squeeze, and cut up the tomatoes.

Expel seeds from the Poblano pepper and finely dice, and daintily cut the green onions. Have the ground cheddar, additional salsa, and sour cream prepared?

When the fluid has vanished from the meat blend, heat the other two tsp. of olive oil in a substantial non-stick skillet over medium-high warmth. (I utilized my preferred 12 Inch Green Pan (offshoot connect).)

If you need to season the oil, include a few stripped garlic cloves and cook just until you smell the garlic, at that point, evacuate. At that point, add the finely diced Poblano chiles and cook 2-3 minutes, just until the peppers begin to mollify.

Include the solidified rice and cook, mix again, for 3-5 minutes or until the cauliflower is warmed through, and any abundance fluid has vanished. (You may need to turn down the warmth a piece, contingent upon how hot your stove gets.)

Mood killer warmth and mix in the cut green onions.

To serve, put a liberal scoop of cauliflower rice in a bowl and top with a scoop of the meat blend.

Include ground cheddar, cut olives, diced avocado, and diced tomatoes.

Serve immediately, with extra salsa and sharp cream to serve at the table whenever wanted.

Any additional hamburger blend and rice can be refrigerated and warmed later if this makes more than you'll eat at once.

Try not to join or add fixings until you're prepared to serve.

NOTES:

Make sure to check the name if you use bought salsa for this formula and pick one that is low in sugar. I utilized Pace Picante Sauce, medium (member connect); however, mild salsa may be better in case you're cooking for kids. If you can't discover solidified cauliflower, utilize my formula for Easy Best Cauliflower Rice with Garlic and Green Onion and saute the cleaved poblano chiles after you evacuate the garlic. Poblanos are regularly called Pacella Peppers in U. S. stores.

wholesome actualities

Protein: 40%

Calories: 20%

Fats: 20%

Low Carb Beef Stroganoff Meatballs

Yield: 4 servings

All-out time: 45minutes

Fixings

- For the meatball blend:
- 1 lb. ground hamburger (80/20)
- One egg
- 1/4 cup almond flour
- 1 tsp fit salt
- 1/4 tsp dark pepper
- 1/2 tsp garlic powder
- 1/2 tsp onion powder
- 1 tsp dried parsley
- 1 tsp Worcestershire sauce
- 2 Tbsp margarine (for singing)
- For the sauce:
- 1 Tbsp margarine
- 2 cups cut mushrooms (white or cremini)
- 1 cup cut onions
- One clove garlic, minced
- 1/2 cups hamburger juices
- 3/4 cup harsh cream
- 1/4 tsp thickener
- salt and pepper to taste
- 2 Tbsp crisp parsley slashed

Guidelines

Join the meatball fixings (aside from the spread) in a medium bowl and blend well.

Structure into 12 meatballs.

Warmth the 2 Tbsp of margarine in an enormous, nonstick saute container.

Cook the meatballs on medium warmth in the margarine until caramelized on all sides and cooked through (2-3 minutes for each team.)

Expel the meatballs from the skillet and put it in a safe spot.

Include the 1 Tbsp of margarine and the 2 cups of cut mushrooms to the skillet.

Cook until the mushrooms are brilliant and fragrant (4-5 minutes.)

Expel the mushrooms from the skillet.

Include the onions and garlic and cook for 3-4 minutes or until relaxed and translucent.

Expel the onions from the skillet.

Add the hamburger juices to your container, and scratch the base to get all the yummy bits off.

Race in your harsh cream and thickener until smooth.

Include the meatballs, mushrooms, onions, and garlic back to the skillet and mix.

Stew on low for 20 minutes.

Season with salt and pepper to taste.

I am trimming with the crisp parsley directly before serving.

Nourishment

Serving Size: (3 meatballs and 1/2 cup sauce Calories: 452Fat: 34g Carbohydrates: 6g net Protein: 24g

Stewing Pot Low Carb Cabbage Roll Soup

Planning time: 20 minutes

Cook time: 3 hours

Absolute Time: 3 hours 20 minutes

Servings: 9

Calories: 356 kcal

Fixings

- 2 tbsp additional virgin olive oil
- Two garlic cloves minced
- 1/2 cup onion cleaved
- 1/2 cup shallots cleaved

- 2 pounds ground hamburger
- 1 tsp dried parsley
- 1/2 tsp dried oregano
- 1 tsp salt
- 1 tsp pepper
- 16 ounces low carb marinara sauce I utilized Rao's image
- 2 cups cauliflower riced
- 5 cups hamburger stock low sodium
- 8 cups cabbage cut

Guidelines

Cook olive oil and garlic over medium-high heat.

Include onions and shallots and cook until mellowed.

Include ground hamburger and cook until sautéed and never again pink.

Add seasonings to hamburger and marinara sauce.

Add the riced cauliflower to the hamburger blend and mix until covered.

Empty the hamburger into the simmering pot.

Empty hamburger stock into the simmering pot and include cabbage.

Mix to join everything.

Cook on high 3 hours or low 6 hours. On the chance that you don't have a stewing pot, mostly cook ground meat in a Dutch broiler or overwhelming soup pot, follow formula and stew on low, secured for about an hour until cabbage is delicate.

Sustenance Facts

Simmering pot Low Carb Un-Stuffed Cabbage Roll Soup

Sum Per Serving   (1.5 cups)

Calories 356 Calories from Fat 234

% Daily Value*

Fat 26g 40%

Immersed Fat 8g 50%

Cholesterol 71mg 24%

Sodium 990mg43%

Potassium 534mg 15%

Sugars 8g 3%

Fiber 2g 8%

Sugar 3g 3%

Protein 20g 40%
Nutrient A 60 1%
Nutrient C 35.1mg 43%
Calcium 60 mg 6%
Iron 2.6 mg 14%

Simmering pot Ground Beef

Planning Time: 10 minutes
Cook time: 4 hours
All out time: 4 hours 10 minutes
Servings: 12
Calories: 209 kcal

Fixings

- 2 cups eggplant cubed
- run salt
- One tablespoon olive oil
- 2 pounds ground hamburger
- Two teaspoons salt
- 1/2 tsp pepper
- 2 tsp Worcestershire sauce
- 2 tsp mustard
- 28 ounces canned diced tomatoes depleted
- 16 ounces canned tomato sauce
- 2 cups mozzarella cheddar ground
- 2 Tablespoons parsley
- 1 tsp oregano

Guidelines

Sprinkle eggplant with a pinch salt and let sit for around 30 minutes. Evacuate into a bowl and mix in olive oil.

Consolidate ground hamburger, salt, pepper, Worcestershire sauce, and mustard. Push on base and sides of a 9×13 slow cooker skillet.

Top meat with eggplant.

Spread tomatoes and sauce over eggplant and add with outstanding fixings.

Cook for 3 hours on low or high 2-3 hours.

Nourishment

Calories: 209kcal
Carbohydrates: 8.1g
Protein: 15.9g

Fat: 12.8g
Sodium: 733mg
Fibre: 2.4g
Gluten-Free Keto Meatloaf
Planning Time: 5 Minutes
Cook Time: 50 minutes
All out Time: 55 minutes
Yield: 1 portion
Fixings

- 2 lbs. grass-nourished 93% lean ground meat
- 2 TBS almond flour
- 2 TBS coconut flour
- 1 tsp garlic powder
- 1 tsp onion powder
- 1 tsp salt
- ¼ tsp pepper
- One egg, gently beaten
- 1 TBS Worcestershire sauce (coconut amines for keto)
- 1 TBS milk (customary, almond and coconut all work)
- ½ cup BBQ sauce (keto endorsed if necessary)

Beating:
½ cup BBQ sauce
Directions
Preheat stove to 3500F Prepare your prospect. You can utilize either a 9×5" portion container or shape into a portion and spot on a rack in an enormous heating sheet (I incline toward the last since it enables any abundance squeezes and fats to deplete)

In a little bowl, combine almond flour, coconut flour, garlic powder, onion powder salt, and pepper. Put in a safe spot.

In an enormous bowl, combine ground hamburger, egg, Worcestershire sauce, milk of decision, and BBQ sauce until consolidated.

Add dry fixings to the meat blend and mix well until joined.

Put your blend into your readied heating container.

Heat at 3500F for 45-65 minutes (time shifts relying upon the thickness of your portion).

Following 20 minutes (part of the way through heating), spread BBQ sauce on the highest point of your meatloaf and return it to the stove to keep cooking until the interior temperature is 1550.

Expel from the oven and let sit for 5 minutes before serving.

Nourishment

Serving Size: Serves 6

Protein 20g

Fat 30g

Calories 50g

Keto Hamburger

Planning Time 20 minutes

Cook Time: 30 minutes

Complete Time: 50 minutes

Servings: 4

Calories: 443 kcal

Fixings

- One huge head cauliflower
- 1-pound ground meat
- One teaspoon cumin
- One teaspoon paprika
- 1/2 teaspoon dried oregano
- Ocean salt and pepper to taste
- 1 cup coconut milk or overwhelming whipping cream
- One bowl of chicken bone soup
- Two eggs
- 1/4 cup cut almonds

Directions

Preheat the stove to 350 degrees.

Cut the cauliflower into florets and dispose of the centre; at that point, cut the cauliflower into considerably littler and progressively uniform pieces.

Spot a steamer pot over medium warmth with a couple of creeps of water, including the cauliflower into the highest and season with salt.

Steam the cauliflower until andante (scarcely cooked) and afterwards expel it from the warmth and put aside revealed.

Spot the ground hamburger in a skillet over medium warmth and season generously with salt and pepper, cumin, paprika, and oregano.

Separate the hamburger into little pieces with a spatula while cooking.

At the point when the meat is generally cooked, expel it from the warmth and put it in a safe spot.

Beat the eggs, cream, and soup together with a spot of salt and pepper in a bowl.

In a dish skillet layer, the cauliflower and ground meat until it is spent.

Pour the egg blend over it, ensuring the meat and cauliflower are secured.

Prepare the goulash for 40 to 45 minutes until the middle is set.

Include the cut almonds and sear for 2-3 minutes.

Let it cool for 5 minutes at that point, serve and appreciate it.

Formula Notes

Net Carbs: 8.7 g

Nourishment certainties dependent on four servings

Nourishment Facts

Sum Per Serving

Calories: 443

Calories from Fat: 241

% Daily Value*

Fat 26.8 g 41%

Starches 16.2 g 5%

Fiber 7.5 g 31%

Protein 39 g 78%

Keto Chili

Planning time: 5 minutes

Cook time: 10 minutes

Complete-time: 15 minutes

Yield: 4 servings

Fixings

- 1 lb. lean ground meat (or turkey)
- 1 tsp ground cumin
- 1 tsp ground coriander
- 1/2 tsp ground cayenne (discretionary)

- 1/2 tsp garlic powder
- 1/2 cup arranged salsa (I utilized Pace Mild)
- salt and pepper to taste

Directions

In a medium pot, join the ground hamburger and the entirety of the flavours.

Cook over medium warmth for around 5 minutes.

At the point when the meat is cooked through, include your salsa.

Stew for 5 minutes.

Discretionary enhancements: red onion, cilantro, avocado, lime, cheddar, sharp cream, corn, peppers

Sustenance

Serving Size: 3/4 cup

Calories: 229Fat: 9g

Sugars: 2g

Protein: 33g

Keto Taco Salad

Yield: 4 salads

All-out time: 25-27 minutes

Planning time: 15 minutes

Cook time: 10-12 minutes

Fixings:

- Serving of mixed greens INGREDIENTS:
- 1 lb. ground hamburger (utilize lean ground meat for South Beach Diet)
- 1-2 tsp. olive oil (varying, for cooking the chicken)
- 2 T Kalyn's Taco Seasoning (or utilize your preferred business taco flavouring)
- 1 cup of water
- 5 oz. child kale leaves washed and spun dry if necessary
- One red chime pepper, cut into slender strips
- 1 cup grape or cherry tomatoes, cut down the middle
- One can (6.5 oz.) cut olives (or if you can't locate the enormous jars of cut olives, cut a container of customary olives)
- 1-2 avocados, diced
- 1 T new pressed lime juice (to hurl with avocado)

DRESSING INGREDIENTS:

- 2 T fresh-squeezed lime juice, see notes
- 1/2 tsp. ground chilli powder, see notes
- 1/4 tsp. ground cumin
- 1/2 tsp. Spike Seasoning (Spike is discretionary, yet it adds enhance. Spike is likely not Keto, so utilize your most loved Keto-affirmed generally useful flavouring on the off chance that you like.)
- 3 T olive oil

Bearings:

Warmth the olive oil in an overwhelming griddle, disintegrate the ground meat into the skillet and cook over medium-high heat until the hamburger is caramelized, breaking separated with a turner as it boils. (I utilize an excellent old potato masher to cut the meat separated!)

At the point when the meat is all around caramelized, sprinkle in the Kalyn's Taco Seasoning (or your taco flavouring) and include the water, mix to consolidate, and stew on low warmth until all the fluid is dissipated, around 8-10 minutes.

At the point when the base of the container is dehydrated, expel the taco meat and let it cool down in a bowl until it's merely somewhat warm.

While the meat cooks, whisk together the 2 T lime juice, ground chilli powder, ground cumin (member interface), Spike Seasoning (offshoot connect) (if utilizing, or another generally useful flavouring), and olive oil to make the dressing.

Wash the infant kale and turn dry if necessary. (I like to clip off the bigger stems. However, it's discretionary.) Cut the red pepper into strips and cut the cherry tomatoes down the middle. Cut the avocado(s) into 3D squares and hurl with the 1 T of lime juice.

Put the kale leaves into a bowl that is sufficiently large to hold all the plate of mixed greens fixings and hurl with the dressing. Include the marginally cooled taco meat, red pepper strips, and tomato parts and hurl once more.

At that point, include the avocado pieces and tenderly hurl once more. (I spare a couple of avocado pieces to embellish every plate of mixed greens.) Serve immediately.

Sustenance

Protein: 50g

Fat: 30g
Calories: 20g
Mexican Zucchini and Beef Skillet
Planning time: 5 minutes
Cook time: 25 minutes
All out time: 30 minutes
Servings: 6 servings
Calories: 315kcal
Fixings
- Two medium zucchinis cut and quartered
- 1/2 pounds ground hamburger
- Two cloves garlic minced
- 10 ounces Mexican style diced tomatoes with green bean stews (salsa or diced tomatoes could be utilized), canned
- One tablespoon bean stew powder
- One teaspoon ground cumin
- One teaspoon salt
- 1/2 teaspoon dark pepper
- 1/2 teaspoon onion powder
- 1/4 teaspoon squashed red pepper drops
Guidelines
Ground meat with minced garlic, salt, and pepper.
Cook over medium warmth until meat is caramelized.
Include tomatoes and remaining flavours. Spread and stew on low warmth for an additional 10 minutes.
Include the zucchini. Spread and cook for around ten additional minutes until zucchini is cooked, yet at the same time, firm.
Sustenance
Serving: 1cup (approx.)
Calories: 315kcal
Carbohydrates: 5g
Protein: 21g
Fat: 23g
Saturated Fat: 9g
Cholesterol: 81mg
Sodium: 498mg
Potassium: 597mg
Fiber: 2g

Sugar: 3g
Vitamin A: 606IU
Vitamin C: 16mg
Calcium: 55mg
Iron: 3mg

Taco Salad Recipe With Ground Beef

Planning time: 10 minutes
Cook time: 10 minutes
All out time: 20 minutes
Servings: 6

Fixings

- 1 lb. ground hamburger
- One teaspoon Avocado oil (or any oil of decision)
- 2 tbsp Taco flavouring (locally acquired or home-made)
- 8 oz Romaine lettuce (cleaved)
- 1/3 cup Grape tomatoes (divided)
- 3/4 cup cheddar (destroyed)
- One medium Avocado (cubed)
- 1/2 cup Green onions (cleaved)
- 1/3 cup Salsa
- 1/3 cup Sour cream

Guidelines

Snap-on the occasions in the guidelines underneath to begin a kitchen clock while you cook.

Heat oil in a skillet over high warmth. Include ground hamburger. Pan-fried food, separating the pieces with a spatula, for around 7-10 minutes, until the meat is seared.

Mix taco flavouring into the ground meat until very much joined.

In the interim, join every single residual fixing in a large bowl. Include the ground hamburger. Hurl everything together.

Nourishment: Nutrition data is evaluated dependent on 85/15 ground hamburger and run of the mill tomato salsa.

Low Carb Lasagna Stuffed Peppers

Planning Time: 14 minutes
Cook Time: 40 minutes
Complete Time: 54 minutes

Fixings

- One substantial red chime pepper

- One huge green chime pepper
- One valuable yellow chime pepper
- One huge orange chime pepper
- 2 ½ cups Tomato Meat Sauce
- 1 cup ricotta cheddar
- 1 cup mozzarella cheddar, destroyed
- ½ cup Parmesan cheddar, ground
- One tablespoon Italian flavouring

Directions

Preheat stove to 400° Line a preparing sheet with aluminium foil.

Cut chime peppers down the middle longwise and evacuate ribs and seeds — spot pepper parts on preparing sheet and heat for 20 minutes on the centre rack.

Expel peppers from the stove. Fill each pepper with ¼ cup tomato meat sauce.

Next, spoon 2 tbsp of ricotta cheddar over the meat sauce in each pepper cup. Pour an extra 1 tbsp meat sauce over the ricotta cheddar.

Top each pepper with 2 tbsp mozzarella cheddar. Prepare on the centre rack for 12 minutes.

Expel peppers from the stove. Top each chilli with 1 tbsp Parmesan cheddar and a sprinkle of Italian flavouring — heat five extra minutes on the top rack.

NOTES

Makes 8 Servings

Per Serving:

Calories: 204

Fat: 11g

Protein: 18g

Net Carbs: 8g

Keto Cheesy Chili Spaghetti Squash Casserole

Yield: 8 servings

All-out time: 40 minutes

Fixings

For the bean stew:

- 1 lb. lean ground hamburger (or turkey)
- 1 tsp ground cumin
- 1 tsp ground coriander

- 1 Tbsp slashed chipotles in adobo (discretionary)
- 1/2 tsp garlic powder
- 1 tsp dried oregano
- 1/2 cup arranged salsa
- salt and pepper to taste

For the goulash

- 4 cups cooked spaghetti squash
- 2 tbsp margarine, dissolved
- 3/4 cup harsh cream
- 1 3/4 cup destroyed cheddar
- slashed cilantro (discretionary)
- sharp cream, salsa, avocado to serve (discretionary)

Guidelines

For the bean stew:

In a medium pan dark-coloured the ground meat prepared with salt and pepper.

Pour off any additional fat and dispose of it.

Include the remainder of the stew fixings and stew for around 10 minutes.

For the dish:

In a medium bowl, consolidate the cooked spaghetti squash and dissolved margarine, hurling to cover.

Season liberally with salt and pepper to taste.

Spread the squash out in a 12 – 14-inch meal dish.

Sprinkle with 3/4 cup of destroyed cheddar.

Spread the sour cream over the cheddar layer.

Spoon on the bean stew and spread it out, leaving a 1-inch outskirt of spaghetti squash around the edge.

Top with the staying 1 cup of destroyed cheddar.

Prepare in a 350-degree stove for 30 minutes or until warmed through.

Sprinkle with cilantro and present with sour cream, salsa, and guacamole or avocado cuts as wanted.

Nourishment

Serving Size: Approximately 1/2 cups

Calories: 284Fat: 20gCarbohydrates: 6g net Protein: 23g

Low Carb Keto Cheese Stuffed Meatloaf

Planning Time: 20 minutes

Cook Time: 45 minutes

Absolute Time: 1 hour 5 minutes
Servings: 12
Calories: 332 kcal
Fixings
- 2.5 pounds of ground meat
- One egg
- 1/2 cup ground parmesan
- 1/2 cup squashed pork skins
- 1/2 tsp salt partitioned
- 1/2 tsp pepper partitioned
- 1/2 tsp garlic powder
- 1/2 tsp onion powder
- 16 ounces solidified defrosted depleted spinach
- 1-1/2 cups destroyed mozzarella cheddar

Directions
Preheat stove to 375 degrees.
In a bowl, blend the ground meat, egg, parmesan, pork skins, 1/4 tsp salt, 1/4 tsp pepper, 1/4 tsp onion powder, 1/4 tsp garlic powder.
Spread this meat blend onto a preparing sheet. Make a ten by 12-inch square shape and around 1/2 inch in thickness.
Uniformly spread out the spinach onto the meat. Sprinkle the staying 1/4 teaspoons of salt, pepper, garlic, and onion powders over the spinach.
Sprinkle the mozzarella over the spinach.
Move up the meatloaf utilizing the material to assist you with turning it over.
Prepare for 40-45 minutes.
Permit to rest around 10 minutes before cutting.
Formula Notes
Net Carbs: 1.3g
Nourishment Facts
Sum Per Serving   (1 g)
Calories 332 Calories from Fat 167
% Daily Value*
Fat 18.6g29%
Soaked Fat 7.6g48%
Cholesterol 117mg39%
Sodium 494mg21%

Starches 2.5g1%
Fiber 1.2g5%
Sugar 0.2g0%
Protein 36.9g74%
Meaty And Cheesy Low-Carb Green Chile Bake
Yield: 8 servings
Planning time: 20 minutes
Cook time: 40 minutes
Absolute time: 1 hour
Fixings
•	One huge 27 oz. can broil and strip green chiles (See note.)
•	4 tsp. olive oil
•	1 lb. ground meat
•	salt and pepper to taste
•	4 cups ground Mexican Blend cheddar (or utilize any gentle cheddar that melts well)
•	One little onion, hacked
•	1 4 oz. can dice green chiles
•	Five eggs
•	1/2 cup sharp cream, at room temperature
•	1/2 tsp. ground cumin
•	1/2 tsp. ground stew powder
•	fixings for filling in as wanted
Directions
Preheat stove to 375F/190C. Shower a 9-inch x 13-inch glass goulash dish with olive oil or non-stick splash. (Any size near that will work.)

Dump the 27 oz. Can green chiles into a colander put in the sink and let them channel.

Warmth 2 teaspoons olive oil in a substantial non-stick skillet over medium-high heat and darker the ground meat well, breaking it separated as it tans.

At the point when meat is very much cooked, season with salt and new ground dark pepper to taste and evacuate it to a plate.

Warmth, the other two teaspoons of olive oil, include the hacked onion and cook until the onions are mollified and beginning to dark-coloured. Include the jar of diced green chiles and juice, mix to join with the onions, and cook 2-3 minutes more. Include the ground hamburger and cook a couple of moments more.

Put the eggs in a small round bowl and beat with a fork to join the whites and yolks. At that point, include the harsh cream, cumin, and bean stew powder and whisk together until the eggs and sharp cream are joined. (It doesn't make a difference if there are a couple of bumps.)

Expel green chiles from the colander in turn and utilize your fingers to open every chile and evacuate any seeds. Spread chiles out on paper towels; at that point, place another layer of paper towel over the top and press down delicately to retain additional dampness.

I like to organize the chiles in two stacks after that so I can partition them equally when I make the layers in the dish.

In the meal dish, make a layer of a large portion of the chiles, a large part of the ground hamburger/onion/chiles blend, and a large portion of the cheddar; at that point, pour over a large portion of the egg blend.

Make a second layer of chiles, meat blend, and cheddar; at that point, pour over the remainder of the egg blend.

Spread the goulash with foil (or a top on the off chance that it has one) and prepare 15 minutes. Cautiously evacuate the thwart and afterwards heat around 25 minutes more, or until the meal is gurgling and the top is pleasantly sautéed.

Serve hot, with additional harsh cream, salsa, or diced avocado to include at the table whenever wanted.

This freezes well and can be warmed in a microwave or a shrouded dish in a toaster broiler or ordinary stove. For best outcomes, defrost in the ice chest before warming.

Sustenance Information:
Yield: 8
Serving Size: 1
Sum Per Serving:
Calories: 461
Total fat: 34g

Saturated fat: 16g
Unsaturated fat: 14g
Cholesterol: 228mg
Sodium: 369mg
Carbohydrates: 6.5g
Fibre: 1g
Sugar: 3g Protein: 33g
Turkey Saltimbocca Meatballs
Yield: 4 servings
total time: 1 hr.
Fixings
•   For the meatballs
•   1 lb. ground turkey (or veal on the off chance that you like)
•   One egg
•   1/3 cup almond flour
•   2 Tbsp ground parmesan cheddar
•   2 Tbsp slashed crude pancetta (or bacon)
•   1 Tbsp slashed new savvy
•   1/4 tsp garlic powder
•   1/2 tsp fit salt
•   1/4 tsp ground dark pepper
•   1 Tbsp olive oil for browning
•   For the sauce:
•   1/4 cup slashed pancetta (or bacon)
•   1/2 cup dry white wine
•   1 Tbsp crisp wise, slashed
•   1/2 tsp lemon juice
•   1/4 tsp garlic powder
•   1 tsp granulated sugar substitute (Swerve and Splenda.)
•   1/4 cup margarine
Guidelines
For the meatballs:

Join the ground turkey, egg, almond dinner, parmesan cheddar, slashed pancetta, hacked sage, garlic powder, salt, and pepper in a medium bowl and blended all together. Form into 12 meatballs. Warmth the olive oil in a nonstick container and cook over medium heat until brilliant dark coloured and cooked through – around 3 minutes for each side. Expel the meatballs from the box and put it in a safe spot.

For the sauce:

Add the pancetta to a similar skillet that you cooked the meatballs in, leaving all the dark-coloured bits in the container (except if it consumed, at that point, start with a new dish.) Cook the pancetta for around 2 minutes or until fresh. Include the white wine, sage, lemon juice, garlic powder, and sugar substitute to the skillet and cook until decreased significantly – around 3 minutes. Include the margarine and speed until softened and the sauce is marginally thickened—season with salt and pepper to taste. Include the meatballs once again into the sauce and mix until very much covered. Serve hot.

NOTES

Approx. nourishment information per serving: 467 calories, 32g fat, 2.5g net carbs, 36g protein

Conclusions

The keto diet has been concentrated widely in little youngsters (some as youthful as three years of age), old populaces, and each period in the middle. Be that as it may, on account of how the keto diet limits carbs so remarkably, it is ideal for screening your social insurance as you are adjusting to the diet.

Yield: 8 servings

At the point when your body begins consuming fat for vitality, it produces ketones (additionally called ketone bodies). You can test your body's degree of ketones to decide if you're in ketosis. During this fat-consuming stage, you can hope to lose a reliable 1-2 pounds every week.

In the underlying phases of a ketosis diet, individuals may feel more worn out and fragile than expected. This weariness happens as the body changes from consuming sugars to consuming fat for vitality. Starches give a snappier explosion of life to the body. So appreciate this diet and get an ideal figure in a matter of moments.